ABSENCE

Your road led through the sea, Your pathway through the mighty waters—a pathway no one knew was there!

—Psalm 77:19 NLT

Dr. Carolyn Lee

Absence
Copyright © 2024 by Dr. Carolyn Lee. All rights reserved.

No part of this publication may be reproduced, stored in a retrieval system or transmitted in any way by any means, electronic, mechanical, photocopy, recording or otherwise without the prior permission of the author except as provided by USA copyright law.

Unless otherwise noted, all scriptures are from THE HOLY BIBLE, NEW INTERNATIONAL VERSION®. Copyright© 1973, 1978, 1984, 2011 by Biblica, Inc.™. Used by permission of Zondervan. Scripture quotations marked (NKJV) are taken from the NEW KING JAMES VERSION®. Copyright© 1982 by Thomas Nelson, Inc. Used by permission. All rights reserved. Scripture quotations marked (NLT) are taken from the Holy Bible, New Living Translation, copyright ©1996, 2004, 2015 by Tyndale House Foundation. Used by permission of Tyndale House Publishers, Carol Stream, Illinois 60188. All rights reserved. Scripture quotations marked (NRSV) are taken from the New Revised Standard Version Bible, copyright © 1989 the Division of Christian Education of the National Council of the Churches of Christ in the United States of America. Used by permission. All rights reserved. Scripture quotations marked TPT are from The Passion Translation®. Copyright © 2017, 2018 by Passion & Fire Ministries, Inc. Used by permission. All rights reserved. ThePassionTranslation.com. Scripture quotations marked MSG are taken from THE MESSAGE, copyright © 1993, 2002, 2018 by Eugene H. Peterson. Used by permission of NavPress, represented by Tyndale House Publishers. All rights reserved. Scripture quotations marked (ESV) are taken from THE HOLY BIBLE, ENGLISH STANDARD VERSION®, Copyright© 2001 by Crossway, a publishing ministry of Good News Publishers. Used by permission.

Published by Agápe Studios. Winona, MN 55987 USA
Cover and Book design: copyright © 2024 by Laurie A. Nelson
www.agapedesignstudios.com All rights reserved.
Interior images: © iStockphoto.com.

Published in the United States of America
ISBN: 979-8-9889805-2-0

The beauty of the book you are holding in your hand is that it will meet you in your grief and walk you back to joy! You will no longer be alone because you will encounter a seasoned friend who has not only walked the lonely, painful path of loss but is delighted to lead you along the path she traveled in finding the Sacred Companion, who led her out of hopeless darkness into the joy-filled hope of the Father's love. The other beauty is that the scriptures buried in the stories will come alive to your heart and you will never read them the same again.

Jim Brackett, Founder/President of Living Loved Ministries Inc.

While absences are real and recurring, no two are the same. Yet, the One who is the same yesterday, today, and forever, is always willing and able to show Himself faithfully present. This is the hope-filled encouragement found in Carolyn's honest and insightful reflections of His care in her own experiences of loss.

Becky Misar, co-author, Journey to the Father

What a beautiful journey through the process of grief and loss. Each devotional tells a story, giving the reader glimpses of the heartache of suffering but also lovingly reminding us to trust in the God who understands our grief and sorrows because He has experienced them Himself. This book will encourage and bring peace to those who are searching for answers.

Reverend Karen Morgan, New Covenant Church, Clyde, NC

As a pastor and counselor for over 30 years, I have personally and professionally walked through grief and loss with a lot of people. Grief is a universal journey we will all take to heal from the deep pain of devastating loss. Sometimes a book is discovered that can put into words what we feel in those lonely and difficult days. This is that book. It will walk with you like a close friend and support you when you need it the most. You will be glad you found this book!

Jim Snider, M. Div., Mind Matters, Wilmington, NC

Thank you, Dr. Lee, for writing this devotional. My heart was gripped by the realness and timeliness of this message. Your vulnerability and transparency will be a source of great strength for those who likewise have suffered deep loss; and, like you, have experienced first hand the suddenness and finality of absence. Isaiah 63:9 says: "In all their affliction He was afflicted." His presence, love and mercy bring redemption and salvation. He will bear us up and carry us throughout the entirety of our life on earth. This devotional is a testimony of what that verse describes. He promises to remain with us and bring about a redemption only He can accomplish.

Dr. David White, Pastor, The Gathering Church, Moravians Falls, NC

*This book is dedicated to
those who need roses in their winter seasons.*

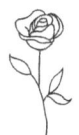

Table of Contents

Missing 1

Promise 4

Jesus+? 7

Dismay 10

Very Present 13

Taken 16

Alive 19

Blooming 22

Gliding 25

Being With 28

The Stranger 31

The Rose 34

Grace 37

Beckoning 39

Rescue 42

Loss 45

No, Nothing 48

Reunion 51

The Towel 54

Confession 56

The Whistle 59

The Room 62

Homestead 65

Bargains 68

Parting 71

Joined	74
The Fog	77
Shelter	80
Turn Right	83
Freedom	86
The Touch	89
God Kind of Faith	92
All In	95
Full Joy	98
This Way	101
Mighty Mite	104
The Squeeze	107
Lost But Found	110
Pop Quizzes	113
Onlies	116
Marked	119
Retreat	122
Break Through	125
Glory	128
One-on-One	131
Abba	134
Identity Theft	137
Coming Home	140
Chaperone	143
Deliverance	146

Missing

Absence can be as simple as the disappearance of a puzzle piece upon the final stages of its assembly. You remember how you selected this puzzle because you liked the promised outcome of the final picture displayed on the front of the box. Spending hours to assemble, your hopes of the beauty of this picture became dashed when you realize one piece is missing.

Questions arise. Did I make a mistake in forcing other pieces together, ones that actually did not fit into that space? I know I'm tempted to force an issue. Did my insistence cause the misplacing of one lone piece? Or did it just drop to the floor? I try to make sense of this incomplete picture.

Life's puzzle pieces may be as simple as a missing cardboard-backed puzzle piece, or it can be as heartbreaking as the absence of a loved one. The anticipated picture of life has been skewed.

Some of life's puzzles come with the lone piece already missing. Something happened on the assembly line. Others are pieces extracted along the way. It may have been my poor choice, or the choice of another. Even some pieces feel as if they've been stolen; like there was some wild conspiracy intended to break our hearts. Life can seem unfair.

Regardless of how the piece or pieces went missing, the vacuum is there. Some thing, or someone, went missing, and the expected life picture is now marred.

Absence is when something or someone is no longer where or as if they usually were. Adjusting to that absence can call for a simple fix or an extreme lifestyle change. Whether it is your misplaced glasses that you are still wearing on top of your head, or the passing of a loved one, there is a heart cry for help. There is an amputation with no prosthesis. God, where are You? you cry. It's for certain that He will never be the absent One. In that we can put our trust.

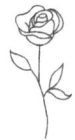
I will never leave you nor forsake you.
—Hebrews 13:5

Father God, my heart is raw from the losses of life. These absences leave me saddened yet You said You would never leave me nor forsake me. Walk me through these hours and days ahead and show me Your tender heart towards me in this time of sorrow. In my weakness, You will be made strong; therefore, I cast my weakness upon You, my God, my strong tower, my ever-present Lord. Amen

---

Reflection:

Promise

The Lord promised He would never leave us. I have to admit my heart is warmed by those words, because I believe that this promise remains forever true. It is in His word. Yet, we are left with the question: How does He fill that vacuum, the very practical outworking of each day, each event, each need of the absent thing or the absent one?

This solitude is far too quiet— far too empty–causing an audible thud made by silence. When heartbreak is so deep, how does He restore the pieces that are missing? When life is in probate, causing a sense of mystery of outcome, how do I make sense of the scattered pieces? Even more baffling is the wonderment of how could the remaining pieces be rearranged to bring purpose.

From ashes He promises beauty. (Isaiah 61:6) Those fine, dusty particles that have been through the fire, are promised to be made into beauty that only He can make. The leftovers of a broken heart, a charred relationship, what could be reshaped from this destruction? The winds of change blow what remains out of our sight, and I scream: how could any of this ever make sense again?

The Three-In-One formed man from mere dust. Our choice now is to hand Them our disintegrated, smoldering ashes and entrust them for the working of beauty. This is surely beyond our understanding. Our only hope is to turn to the One who is the Maker of all things, the restorer of that which is lost, and the One to heal the broken hearts.

Bewilderment leaves us in a place of confusion or disorientation. In our own limitations, we are unable to fix what is broken. We come face to face with our weakness and therefore our need for the only One who can make sense of all that has happened. He explains Himself through the prophet Isaiah:

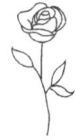
For My thoughts are not your thoughts; neither are your ways My ways, declares the Lord...so is My word that goes out from My mouth: it will not return to Me empty, but will accomplish what I desire and achieve the purpose for which I sent it. You will go out with joy and be led forth in peace.... —*Isaiah 55:9, 11-12*

Father, Your word gives me hope in the midst of my trials and testings. I run to it, I throw myself into what You say is the fruit of such abandonment. I'm learning to trust Your promises and Your presence regarding every absence of my life. Amen

---

Reflection:

Jesus + ?

There are times when the Spirit of God will speak something to us when we were not fully aware we were asking. Then again, maybe we had asked when we simply cried, 'Help!" And He chose to answer that cry in a particular way.

Driving to church one morning, preparing my heart for His presence, I heard Him ask: "Am I not enough?" Along with His words came what He permitted me to feel of His heart. There seemed a sadness tucked in that question. A sadness that, after all of His attempts to assure us of His shepherding our lives, we still anticipate we need 'Jesus + something.'

Given the absence of something or someone so dear to our hearts, it is so easy to feel that life would be more satisfying if He would just fix what's broken, replace what's missing, fill what's so empty...Then, embarrassed, I say: "Oh, by the way, do add Yourself, Lord!"

Again, He says, "Am I not enough?" That question arrests my thoughts and convicts my heart because I can so easily 'pseudo-bargain' with God to fill my void. He reminds me of why the Trinity divinely planned my entry into this life: to have fellowship with Him. "Even before He made the world, God loved us and chose us in Christ to be holy and without fault in His eyes. God decided in advance to adopt us into His own family by bringing us to Himself through Jesus Christ. This is what He wanted to do, and it gave Him great pleasure." (Ephesians 1:4-5 NLT)

So, before the absences took place in my life, I was already chosen for Him. He expects to be my First Love. I stray so easily when I feel that He would be enough, if only…. (fill in the blank)

His poignant question stirs my heart. We admit to ourselves that we are prone to bargain with Him, to present before Him that which we feel would cause us more peace and joy.' Jesus +' is our natural bent. The only way out of this self-imposed confinement is to lean heavily into Him: the One who is more than enough! El Shaddai, the covenant Hebrew name through which God reveals Himself means 'the all-sufficient One,' or 'the God who is more than enough.'

He is not just the God of yesterday; He is the God of now. He is not the God of 'someday I'll be enough.' No, He said, "I AM." I am El Shaddai!

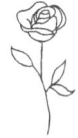 …God loved us and chose us…. —*Ephesians 1:4b NLT*

Father, You deliver us and set us on high. When we call on You, You answer and are with us in trouble. You have promised to satisfy us with long life and to show us Your salvation. Help us to trust You more, regardless of the missing pieces of life. Amen

Reflection: _____

Dismay

We had loved each other as friends, spending hours together over 52 years. Now, her 99 senior years were coming to a close. We had planned for this day, as best we could, by rehearsing her favorite scripture, trying to prepare for when that time would come. Father God did not disappoint, for grace was her crown that evening of her departure.

She and I came to understand that the adversary targets our vulnerable places and attempts to break down our courage. He moves in the areas of sadness that are fed by fears of that which seems unpleasant. My friend and I had prayed one of the key words in her favorite Bible passage: that she would not 'dismay." This timely scripture in Isaiah 41:10 reads: "So do not fear, for I am with you; do not be dismayed, for I am your God. I will strengthen you and help you; I will uphold you with My righteous right hand."

The prefix 'dis' means to experience an emotional breakdown of courage. It puts a negative spin on a situation. Yet, His word strengthened her as well as myself: "Do not be DISmayed." The remaining portion of the word is 'may.' This means the ability to do something. We see that, within this one word depicts the conflict of the soul–the fight between a negative spin and the God-given ability to be strong. Isaiah prophesied God's strength would forever stand the test of time: "For I am your God."

I witnessed the absence of my friend's last breath as His righteous right hand took her Home. I had promised, given His grace, that I would be there with her, and that she would not be 'dismayed.'

It seemed as if she waited for me to arrive; for in less than an hour, she went to be with Him.

Preparing to officiate her memorial service, I wondered what I was going to do with this void. How would I face the absence of my dearest friend to whom I ran when I wanted to share my joys, my sorrows, and much laughter over our 'inside' jokes. We shared many births, weddings and departures in both families. With whom would I feel safe, safe enough to share my feelings and that I would never hear: "I told you so"? What friend could share in my devotion to Jesus—the centerpiece of my life—in ways like we had? With whom could I replace the summary of such unconditional love between friends?

The Lord comforted me as I pondered these questions. On the day of her service, I shared my final remarks: "Whether mansion neighbors or not, I will find you when I get to Heaven. I will then be able to tell you everything that's happened since your absence, and I can do so for all eternity." He turned my friend's 'dis' into 'may' by fulfilling His promised word. Now I lean into "His righteous right hand" to uphold me in adjusting to her absence.

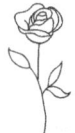
> ...fear not, for I am with you; be not dismayed, for I am your God; I will strengthen you, I will help you, I will uphold you with my righteous right hand.
>
> —Isaiah 41:10 ESV

Father, relationships can be nearly as close as blood kin. Those with whom we bond can inhabit a place in our hearts that, upon losing, can leave crevices in the soul. Only You can fill those voids with promises that You will uphold us when become fainthearted. Scoop us up into Your arms and comfort these tender places, Lord. Amen.

Reflection:

Very Present

I had not known Jim long as we had just been introduced through mutual friends. Our short time together was centered around Jesus, my favorite subject. Jim remembered that time together when he called one morning out of concern for his secretary. She was bound by trauma and just sat at her desk, staring into space.

"Would you come? She needs help!" My reply was immediate as I promised to arrive within the hour. Then my thoughts challenged: "What do you think you are going to do to fix her?" Immediate prayers went up for the Lord's guidance. His response brought one scripture to mind: "God is our refuge and strength, a very present help in trouble." (Psalm 46:1 ESV) That was all I heard; so I trusted it would be all that was needed.

As I arrived at the business office, Jim ushered his secretary and myself into the private conference room. It was the first time I had met this woman. I was convinced that chatty conversation was not in order for this troubled one. Having known she had witnessed a man having a sudden heart attack leading to death at a meeting the week before, I knew she was replaying the scene in her mind. I read to her the scripture the Lord had given to me. Then I asked this question: "Since He is a very present help, how long did it take for the Lord to be on the scene to help this man at the end of his life?" She thought about it a moment, and then answered, "A very present help means He was there even before it happened!"

I replied, "Yes! It did not take Him by surprise. He went before him and was very present."

She exclaimed, "I GOT IT!" She received the revelation of God's presence, and all trauma was lifted. It was gone! In less than 10 minutes in this private conference room, the word of God went deeply into her soul and absorbed all traumatic memories of the sudden absence of her business associate.

Cheerful conversation and freedom over our lunch together with Jim were indicators that this woman had been set free. Jim, still in amazement at the short amount of time it took, witnessed transformation. My only reply was: "The word of God works! That's all He gave me. And that was all that was needed."

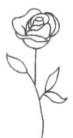 God is our refuge and strength, a very present help in trouble. —*Psalm 46:1 ESV*

Father, Your word is powerful. It is able to turn on light in the midst of darkness. Your word goes into the deepest recesses of our hearts and restores what has otherwise paralyzed us. Life begins to flow again in the places where You have spoken Your truth and make Your presence known. Amen.

Reflection:

Taken

These words came to me from Holy Spirit: "Tell My people that I am territorial." Whoa! That word 'territorial' had always had a negative meaning to me. It seemed like some person was possessive either with space or with relationship, demanding their rights over mine. Yet, I knew Holy Spirit was never negative in thought nor in what He wanted to accomplish.

He reminded me that believers in Jesus Christ belong to Him. The word of God explains that we are sealed as His, we are His workmanship. He fashioned us in purpose before the foundation of the world. Therefore, He had every right to claim His territory. (Ephesians 4:30; 2:10; 1:4)

Then He added: "Tell My people that, as My betrothed, they are to proclaim these words:

"I AM TAKEN!"

He continued that there would be 'proposals' coming from the world, the flesh, and the devil. These so-called proposals would vie for our affection, and they would seek to betroth themselves to us. These 'proposals' would easily fit right into absences, those voids within our souls, where we had suffered losses, offenses, disappointments, heartaches; all resulting in distrust. Something would fill that vacuum.

When Father, Son and Holy Spirit saw formless void, the absence of life, God spoke to that vacuum and brought forth life. He betrothed

Himself to this space and filled it with Himself. That remains true for all believers: to betroth ourselves to the One who formed the earth and all that is within it, the One who hovers over us, calling us to know that we are His.

I am taken!

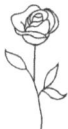 In the beginning God created the heavens and the earth. Now the earth was formless and empty, darkness was over the surface of the deep, and the Spirit of God was hovering over the waters. —*Genesis 1:1-2*

Father, I ask for Your daily grace to remember that I belong to You, even in times of great loss. I am Yours, and You are mine. "We walk together as good friends should and do. We clasp our hands, our voices ring with laughter." ("My God and I," by Austris Whithol, 1971)

Reflection:

Alive

"Regardless of faith or status, we cannot avoid loss. It is inevitable. The questions remain:

Will I walk with God as he teaches me how to deal with it? Or will it be a crippling agent? Will I glean the deeper life lessons? Will I walk away from God, or will I run to Him?"

This quote is copied from my book *"Seamless: Always and Forever,"* the story of the bountiful grace of God shown to me from the day we learned of our son Patrick's battle with cancer to the day of his departure.

The journey with our son throughout his illness, witnessing his valiant fight of faith to the day of his entry into Heaven stirred up raw emotions in all of us who knew and loved him. They would rage as we lost him slowly, and very painfully, to the cruelty of disease. An absence came that shook our family to its core. A vibrant, young man, who brought such joy to so many, was taken Home so early. Way too early for us to grasp.

The choice remained. How would we walk through this gut-wrenching grief while still trusting in the goodness of God? Did we still believe He is the Healer? Would we hang tight to our hope that we would reunite one day on the other side? His absence begged for words to explain how we felt. None would come.

In such a surprising way, a time came when I could begin to breathe deeply again. Grief is a strange thing, with a mind of its own.

And the journey to recovery is unique for every person. Shopping at a local store, I met an acquaintance whom I had not seen in several years. As we updated about our families, I asked if she had known Patrick died? Immediately Holy Spirit resounded: "He is NOT dead!" I was stunned, yet my Bible knowledge grounded my understanding of what He meant. So I promised Him, and myself, that I would meditate more on Patrick's seamless journey to Heaven, who is very much alive, as opposed to the morbid concept of death and great void.

Patrick's absence from his body left a vast void in our family. At the same time, his faith in Jesus Christ as Savior assured him of relocation from earth to Heaven. My outlook changed as I was able to imagine his time away from us, while so very present with his Lord. The joys began to seep into my soul in place of such foreboding sorrows. Heaven's reality came even closer because of my boy being there. His absence is now being filled with the hope of eternal life, both for him and for me and my family who will reunite one day. We will never again experience absence.

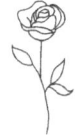 When the perishable has been clothed with the imperishable, then the saying that is written will come true: Death has been swallowed up in victory.
—I Corinthians 15:54

Father, salvation through Jesus Christ promises us eternal life. Scriptures promise that, once we have accepted Jesus as Savior, we are secured and will never die a spiritual death. Though the body perishes, we remain alive and are given an imperishable body. Thank You for saving my son's soul and making Yourself known to Him. He is ALIVE with You forever. Amen

Reflection:

Blooming

The retreat title was "Consider the Lily." As I prepared the message, I was prompted to buy lily bulbs for each of the women attending. This served as a visual of the journey: that this ugly, hairy bulb would transform into an item of beauty.

My son was in the battle for his life from the horrors of cancer and chemotherapy. So, with all the faith I could muster, I grabbed hold to the belief that the ugliness of the lily bulb would come to express its contents of a beautiful life. Still, how could something so ugly turn into something so lovely as these lily bulbs promised? Life is within, I rehearsed

The bulb had to go through a process of breakdown in order to release its tiny stems of hope. As God designed it, the planted bulb represented our desperate hope for our son's recovery. I trusted it would assure us of the floral wonder. Time and again, this tender stem would face the dark ceiling of earth's soil. What courage God placed within that baby stem to glare at its goliath-like, dirt ceiling with commanding faith of breakthrough.

The journey was arduous as our son's tiny faith stem, being pressed so hard on all sides, courageously pushed against that demanding soil. That rebellious dirt insisted on remaining undisturbed. At the same time, Patrick fought against the taunting soil. When the retreat was ended, I said to our son, with unwavering faith, "The lily DOES bloom!" It's written in nature, I reminded him, while I also reminded myself.

Yes, the lily did make its way to beauty. I am left with imagining what my son's appearance is now. I know that he 'blooms' in his relocation, with no toiling, no spinning, and in full glorified beauty.

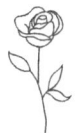 Consider the lilies of the fields, how they grow: they neither toil nor spin; yet I tell you, even Solomon in all his glory was not dressed like one of them.

—Matthew 6:28-33 NLT

Father, the lily does bloom, as You promised. Its struggle is real, yet You designed it to bring forth beauty in its time. You journey with us, never leaving nor forsaking Your own. May we never lose hope that Your eternal plan will always produce the promised hope. Amen.

Reflection: _____

Gliding

Grief's journey can be a strange one, being quite different per person. For those of us who are prone to ask 'why' or 'how' to master emotions, we work tirelessly at trying to find grief's proverbial 'handle.' Most of us long to prevent its rebellious outbursts, the ones that blindside us, especially in front of others.

The Hospice chaplain looked at me, knowingly, as I explained to her how important it was for me to be strong, to carry myself with grace. After all, I had many responsibilities to oversee.

I could not afford to break down. Such was MY plan. In retrospect we come to learn that grief is the equivalent of love. The deeper we have loved, the deeper we grieve. Emotions cannot always be controlled, especially those that erupt without permission. They tantrum themselves, one way or the other, in fits of rage, sulkiness, or alas: the ugly cry.

In this journey, there are metaphors written in nature that speak a language that is understandable. The swan was introduced to me as a symbol of grief. These elegant creatures appear to glide about the waters with no effort. Their graceful posture implies that they have not a care in the world. Yet, with a closer look, they teach us otherwise.

Underneath the waters, their legs and webbed feet propel them forward. Their wings are partially opened to bring balance and efficiency in movements. Heads and necks are used to thrust them forward in the watery pool. Their exercised muscles enable their bodies to work their way through the wet pathway with elegance.

Grief teaches us that there is a balance between emotional release and the God-given grace to go forward. Though our soul's 'webbed feet' may be out of sight, they are paddling hard to make it— one little swim at a time. It's impossible for human efforts to be the master of this journey, for grief demands authenticity.

Just as it is with the swan's head and neck in its kick-start, without the mind and will being immersed in the waters of God's word, this 'little swan' would not gain the unction to move forward. Though we may have tried to fool others of our own smooth moves, while hiding our sorrows, the Creator knows each intricate aspect of our soul. Gliding along with the Spirit of God as our lead, dipping frequently into the waters of His word, we will be enabled to face tomorrow's predictable absences.

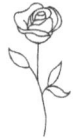

> But He said to me, My grace is sufficient for you, for My power is made perfect in weakness. Therefore I will boast all the more gladly about my weaknesses, so that Christ's power may rest on me. —*2 Corinthians 12:9*

Father, Your grace propels us forward into the paths of life when we lean into You. Though our flesh will paddle furiously at times of emptiness and void, it is in those times we realize how much more we need to trust in Your power and nearness. Amen

Reflection: _____

Being With

The air was thick. All of my senses were stirred as we entered the city limits of my husband's hometown. I took several deep breaths as landmarks seemed to tower over me, taller than ever. Coastal atmosphere was pungent with familiar smells of a fisherman's paradise.

Nearly two years had gone by since my husband passed. Yet it seemed that time was lying to me. Our honeymoon at the beach hotel, the births of four babies and the visual of our car bulging with baby necessities, crowded my mind defied time's advancement. Countless holiday reunions and beach vacations had filled our fifty-five years of marriage. The mental photo album flashing in my mind nearly brought me to my knees. Having my youngest daughter and two of my granddaughters with me assisted in this first trip back to the hometown. In my husband's absence, it felt a bit disloyal for me to be there without him leading the way.

Those of us in the car were undoubtedly watching each other. A loving husband, a doting father, and a proud PawPaw was absent. So we clothed ourselves in bravery, tucking away the tender feelings while aware of this void. Pretending we could make it through without leaking emotional streams was going to be a challenge.

By this time in my grief journey, I had learned that 'being with' was one of the dearest gifts to offer when someone is suffering heartache. Many friends had asked for understanding in how to offer their comfort. Being honest with me, some admitted they stayed away out of fear of upsetting me. Others said they did not know what to say. Still others repeated some of the most-used "bereavement comments," only to realize their words fell to the ground.

No doubt everyone means well. We may sadly fail at touching the heart that aches. The grieving one may need to talk; then again, they may not. By offering the gift of 'being with,' we may learn what is most effective. Knowing there is an absence, our presence just may help to soothe the raw wounds. Giving space, where space is most needed, is also a way of 'being with.'

Some of my dearest memories are of those who sat quietly beside me. I can still remember the surprise when one drove ten hours to visit a short time and then turn around to drive back home. A promise was made by a friend that I would never go to bed again without hearing her say 'goodnight' to me. Years later, this offer still stands. There is the one who texted me regularly for the first few years, assuring me of prayers on my behalf, while insistent that I need not reply. All efforts, even the ones unmentioned, caused my aching heart to feel these kind souls were 'being with.'

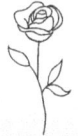 Finally, all of you should be of one mind. Sympathize with each other. Love each other as brothers and sisters. Be tenderhearted, and keep a humble attitude.

— *1 Peter 3:8 NLT*

Father, thank You for sending those You choose to comfort us in times of sorrow and loss. May we forgive those who did not know how to comfort us. Help us to forgive those who tried and missed touching those raw absences. You were there and never failed us. Amen

Reflection:

The Stranger

The promise was kept as we headed for the beach with my granddaughters. A spot was chosen where we could fit ourselves among the crowded beach towels; so we positioned our surf chairs at the water's edge. My senses were heightened at the smell of the salty ocean air. The movement of the tide rehearsed memories of vacations at this beach. At times my grieving emotional tide would be low, and I could see things a bit more clearly. At other times, the tide of emotions came in with a fierceness that blinded me from seeing anything else but my husband's absence. I learned, as time passed by, to hold on when the tide was high, knowing it would come to an ebb once again. For months, this is how I had learned to counsel myself throughout the day.

Facing the ocean's horizon, I reflected upon the scope of our years together. My daughter and I talked of happy memories at this surf side. I shared details of her grandparents' early days, celebrating their big-band era at the aging pier. Memories flooded our minds as family history spoke volumes and chronicled gratitude for God's goodness. Peering into my eyes, my daughter asked, "Mom, are you glad that you came here, your first time back without Dad?" I said, quite honestly, "I have mixed feelings. I'm delighted to be here with the three of you; yet I admit to the need to breathe deeply just to keep my emotions in check." She squeezed my hand and offered her presence: the most precious gift that was needed.

Father God will sometimes use the darkest backdrops to set into place His brightest light. I could not have anticipated the miracle would happen next. An older man, a stranger, who had been out swimming in the ocean, came walking out of the water and straight towards me. He had a red rose in his hand. As he approached me, I admit to being leery of his intent; but he said to me: "I was out swimming, and I saw this rose. I knew I was to give it to you." Then he walked away.

Stunned by this encounter, my daughter and I stared at each other in disbelief. My two granddaughters came running out of the water approaching us, questioning: "What just happened? Why did this man give you this red rose?" I was unable to answer, perplexed at why this stranger came directly to me, out of all the people lined upon the beach this Labor Day weekend.

As the family re-entered the ocean to swim, I sat in my water's-edge chair and pondered: "What are the odds that a rose would be found amidst the turbulent ocean's breakers, in tact, in spite of the salty waters? How could its petals still be in place, its leaves attached? Why was this rose specifically assigned to me?" I spent the rest of the day and evening pondering these questions.

It was the next morning that both granddaughters announced to me their conclusion, "This was an angel."

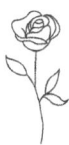 Don't forget to show hospitality to strangers, for some who have done this have entertained angels without realizing it! —*Hebrews 13:2 NLT*

Father, You make pathways where we least expect them, and You manifest Your love at a time when it is most needed. Thank You for touching my heart and the hearts of my family in such a miraculous way. Amen.

Reflection: _____
_____
_____
_____
_____
_____
_____
_____
_____
_____
_____
_____

The Rose

A rose. A real rose, undisturbed, and special delivery just to me.

I remain amazed at God's goodness. Reenacting every detail of this miraculous event, I tried to make sense of it. How did this rose get into the ocean in the first place? How did it survive the breakers where my granddaughters and this stranger had been swimming? Every petal. Every leafy branch in place. How did this man know to bring it to me?

My youngest granddaughter explained that she had seen this man swimming nearby until he submerged into the waters. She told us that her concern was that he had drowned. But she reported that he came up out of the churning salty waves with this rose in his hand. She watched as he swished away through the waves and approached me on the beach.

"The secret things belong to the Lord our God, but the things that are revealed belong to us and to our children forever...."
—Deuteronomy 29:29

I sought understanding. This rose, without any doubt in my mind, nor the minds of my loved ones, had been a supernatural gift sent to me by my Heavenly Father at a time when my emotions churned like the ocean's breakers. Up from life's turbulence came a blessing that I would not have even had faith to pray for.

My head was barely above my own emotional waters, yet He was there. Apostle Peter came to mind as he cried out to Jesus while sinking into the stormy waves. Our loving Father knows what we need and when we need it. This red rose spoke of His compassion for the absence I was experiencing. In the midst of turmoil and heartache, He sees us. And the measure of His compassion is beyond the vastness of that great ocean. The ocean He made. We are never beyond His reach. Nor is He limited by our circumstances.

Another glance at this gift from Him and I see that there are no thorns, nor even thorn buds, on the long green stem. Research revealed that there are very few thornless roses. Most hybrids have at least a few thorns. Nevertheless, my rose, the one chosen by Him, delivered by an angel, reminded me that Jesus painfully bore a crown of thorns upon His brow (John 19:2). Bearing the suffering, He was greatly humiliated. My thornless rose told me that He understood how the absence of my husband hurt me, and that is why He bore my sorrows Himself.

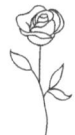

Your path led through the sea. Your way through the mighty waves; a pathway no one knew was there.
—*Psalm 77:19 NLT*

Father, Your paths walk through walls, hardened hearts, broken dreams, and through the ocean waters. Help me to never doubt Your ability to break through any barrier that causes me to feel apart from You. Amen.

Reflection:

Grace

Oh the wonders in the arrival of God's 'special delivery.' So unexpected. I placed the rose in the wet sand beside my beach chair so it could have a continual drink. Standing tall, the rose announced its love message. Foamy refreshment came from the shallow ocean waters that surrounded its beauty. The stranger walked by once more and advised: "Take care of it; the salt water is not good for it." Then he was gone. My young granddaughter later remarked she had seen him approach me again, "then he was gone."

Dinner time was nearing so we began packing our things. Suddenly, to our amazement, a very large wave, away from its tidal basin, drenched my daughter and me. Our clothes, towels, and cell phones caught the downpour. We stared at one another as we wondered how this happened at the shallow water's edge. My granddaughter was the first to see that the rose had been ejected from its wet, sandy vase. The large wave had propelled it down the beach by the force of tide. She ran after it. How relieved I was to have it retrieved and placed back in my care.

Later that evening, I heard the Spirit of God say: "You felt as if a rogue wave had taken your husband away; but, today, grace brought you his love." (My young granddaughter's name is Gracie.)

Philip Yancey writes: "Grace, like water, flows to the lowest part." In times of despair and loneliness, Father touches our hearts and writes a fresh new message of hope.

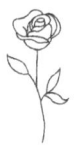 And He has generously given each one of us supernatural grace, according to the size of the gift of Christ. —*Ephesians 4:7 TPT*

Father, You never cease to understand our deepest needs. Though the waters of life can be turbulent and disruptive, Your grace is always sufficient. You make a way in the midst of some of our most disturbing times and redeem the moments we submit to You. Amen.

Reflection:

Beckoning

Absence is the vacuum left by something expected or wanted, yet no longer present. The wounds that cut deep into the soul are determined by the value placed on what is missing. Misplaced keys can be aggravating; but nothing compares to the loss of a meaningful relationship. Death is a part of life, and we are warned we must be prepared for the reality. But how could we be shored up for the voids that it brings?

Trying to adjust to the absence of my life partner was difficult. Every aspect of life begged for his presence. Family occasions were pock-marked by the empty chair. Nights seemed darker than usual, and the creaking sounds of the house were haunting. Family photos were slimmer with a son and a husband no longer wrapping their strong arms across our shoulders.

The voice of the Spirit called out as I drove to church one morning: "Am I not enough?" I felt the sadness of His heart as I felt lured to His side as He called me into a deeper intimacy than ever before. My wounded heart still longed for my missing loved ones. I loved the Lord with all my heart—or at least I thought I did. Was He offering me a relationship that was going to satisfy this breaking heart, I pondered. I had heard of others who had found this deeper walk with Him; however, it sure felt different when it became my own.

Grace filled my heart at times; then I would feel Him nearby. But, in order to wholeheartedly throw myself into His loving arms, to entrust Him with every cry, every ache, the agonizing vacancy of social singleness, I had to know that He would be that for me. Holy spirit said, "I miss you." I heard that tender voice somewhere in the midst of my busyness—doing those things I had chosen to fill the empty voids. Again, His voice would call and I would rush off to fulfill a duty. "Do you trust Me?" He beckoned. I could see that I was going to be facing the idols of my heart; those people whom I had left fill those places. The thought of releasing them fully felt so disloyal to their memories. Yet...where else would I go?

Simon Peter faced this question when some of the disciples he had walked with began to vanish. Jesus asked Peter what he would do if He ascended from where He had once come from? Peter replied, "To whom else would we turn? You have words of eternal life." Peter faced the same sorrowful challenge: what would he do if Jesus was no longer on earth? (John 6:60-68 NKJV)

My question remained: Can my God touch the heart wrenching needs that agitate my soul? Was it possible to walk with Holy Spirit and to know Him as my closest companion, my guide, and to be my intimate prayer partner?

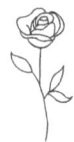

As the Father has sent Me, so I send you. And when He had said this, He breathed on them and said to them, Receive the Holy Spirit. —*John 20:20-21 NLT*

Father, my answer came. I had to simply receive from Holy Spirit. Help me to remember that You sent Holy Spirit to walk within me and beside me throughout my life. Being my companion and guide, He touches my soul at some of the loneliest times. Never does He leave me, as promised. You are more than enough! Amen.

Reflection:

Rescue

A five-hour layover in Heathrow Airport in London would not have been so bad except I privately pouted over a missed tour of London. As a mission's team leader, I settled down for the anticipated wait. It seemed as if every nation and tribe hustled to meet their flights. My eyes focused to my left on a small girl, no older than six. The hurried passengers towered over her slight build while her face was showing distress. Studying the details of the situation, I wondered why no one was aware of her being alone—alone with mounting fear. She was lost in the crowd, and strangers were way too busy to notice. Her features revealed that she was from India. So I watched her, as she passed nearby our area. Then, one more look at this child's panic-stricken face and I knew I had to go to her. I advised my husband that I would be back–a child needed my help. I hoped that he heard me as I rushed to her.

A foreigner approaching could have been frightening to the child, so I smiled and spoke in the softest voice I could muster. An obvious language barrier lay between us, but she read my attempts as I hand-gestured questions about her parents. She let me know she could not search for them with limited view, so, with permission, I lifted her in my arms. My voice intonation and facial expressions would be our way to communicate as a 'game' was now in order. My tone persuaded her that I was not worried and that we would 'play' until we found her mom and dad. Indian adults would pass us by, and I would smile and ask if they were hers. Refusing to reveal distress, I carried her back and forth three times the entire length of the airport lobby. Her parents were nowhere to be seen.

Desperate for help, I approached a kiosk and was thrilled to know the female clerk spoke English. To my advantage, we were able to talk about the seriousness of the situation. The clerk reported that, in her years of experience, several children had been left at the airport, intentionally. Abandoned. Left alone in the absence of any adult supervision. The clerk and I walked with the child a little while longer, pretending to play 'the game' while we both prayed that this was not our situation.

After one more walk the length of the lobby, we agreed to publicly announce that a child was missing her parents and could be found at the service desk. This had not been the clerk's first choice, advising abductors could pose as a distant relative, snatching the child. Perching my little friend upon the counter, I observed her desperate plea. Holding her little hands in mine, I continued to smile, playing our pretend 'game' until she connected with her family. Some of the hurried passengers were now interested in what was happening. They gathered around the service desk, waiting and hoping to see a reunion. A frantic Indian man squeezed his way through the crowd and ran towards us. Tears cascaded from his eyes as he neared his baby girl. Joy and tears erupted from us all, as this man, who spoke no English, gestured to me the enormity of his gratitude. Just before they left, he asked the child to turn towards me and thank me. She shook her head 'no.' She didn't want to look my way. I had been the face that reminded her of her father's absence, I understood she needed that vacuum filled and didn't ever want to look back.

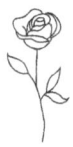 ...But one thing I do, forgetting those things which are behind and reaching forward to those things which are ahead, I press toward the goal... — *Philippians 3:14*

Father, we are never out of Your sight. You are our rescue when we are lost. How precious is Your shepherding care–never out of reach. Amen.

Reflection:

Loss

He always made me laugh. Even his portly belly would jiggle as he watched me laugh at his silliness. Uncle James and his family joined us many Sundays after church for a meal. I hardly remember the menu because the laughter was center stage. He loved the Lord and spent many road trips spreading the gospel wherever he was invited. It was a joy to share our faith together. I smile as I remember those wonderful occasions. Then came the diagnosis.

ALS was new to my family. We had never witnessed its ravages upon one's body. It took its toll and rendered him unable to do normal functions, to communicate, and to laugh again. Towards his latter days on earth, the most he could do was bat his eyelids once or twice to indicate 'yes' or 'no' responses to our questions.

The absence of joy, the presence of disease, can halt one's life and deeply affect those around them. I longed to see his belly jiggle up and down again, for him to tell me another cute joke, but his belly had diminished in size while his soul no longer carried his infectious humor. My youngest daughter played a psaltery as her home schooling music interest. She practiced Uncle James' favorite songs and played them for him at bedside. Tears flowed though the rest of his face could not testify to his emotions. The tender sounds of the psaltery, played by his great niece, was a gift that traveled beyond words. His life was cut short and our lives were deeply affected by his absence.

Diane was known for her infectious laughter. Her favorite source of humor was herself. She told it all: ugly and pretty. Nothing held back, no matter how shocking. Our group of friends had years of fellowship and hilarity. She told of hiding the cartons of ice cream in the bushes before arriving home, as if removal of evidence could affect her weight. She played tricks on others in ways that most people would not even think of. She loved deeply and cried easily when one of her friends was in pain. All of this and more was my friend Diane. Her life was cut short, to be ended by another diagnosis of ALS.

There are others who have suffered or are suffering this horrible disease. Lou Gehrig was the first most of us heard of having such a devastating diagnosis: one that brings muscle and nerve nourishment to an end. Thus the illness bore his name: The Lou Gehrig Disease. It ended his life in 1941, halting the career of one of baseball's most beloved players. He played for the New York Yankees for 17 years and was called "The Iron Horse" due to his ability to play baseball despite suffering from a variety of injuries. He was 36 years old at diagnosis and 62,000 people witnessed his final speech at retirement.

This is not the only disease that creates absence. Most every reader of this book could testify to the huge loss suffered at the passing of a loved one. Some may even be fighting a health battle themselves. Loss is loss. Absence of health is not only limiting but can sometimes end a life long before it is considered 'time to go Home.'

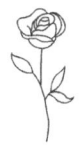 **I will never leave you nor forsake you.** —*Hebrews 13:5b*

Father, You know. You see. And You promise to reveal Yourself in the midst of some of the darkest times. Amen.

Reflection:

No, Nothing

Over the course of my life, especially as a pastor and Hospice chaplain, I have witnessed the sufferings of countless ones whose health was failing. Many have gone through declines that would challenge the strongest of believers. Yet, I have also witnessed those who had faith that refused to yield to fear.

I told my son, as he fought cancer, that he was my 'hero.' His reply was: "No, Mom, I'm just trying to make it through while I'm certain that Jesus has me in His hands." I watched him fulfill his sportsman bucket list when most people would have succumbed to the bed. Not him. He talked, walked, hunted, and witnessed for Jesus. And seldom if ever complained. In his final days, he bought ice cream for all the nurses on the hospital hall. Heroism can be defined in many ways. American Heritage Dictionary calls it: the display of courage, bravery, fortitude, and unselfishness. As his mama, I imagine his picture posted right beside the word 'hero.'.

Absence of health begs for the presence of the Lord's grace. Many are able to realize this amazing grace. They are sources of inspiration to all who surround them. No doubt we would wish things to be different. No one welcomes such sorrow and suffering.

As a friend was declining in health, I learned of his diagnosis. Disease had struck once again, and my heart ached for even another to be going Home–so soon. Then I heard these words: *"Nothing separates Me from my child."*

Nothing? *"No, nothing!"*

The Apostle Paul, who had suffered much torment in his life, wrote to the church at Rome:

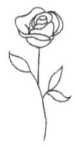 I am convinced that nothing can ever separate us from God's love. Neither death nor life, neither angels nor demons, neither our fears for today nor our worries about tomorrow—not even the powers of hell can separate us from God's love. No power in the sky above or in the earth below—indeed, nothing in all creation will ever be able to separate us from the love of God that is revealed in Christ Jesus our Lord. —*Romans 8:38-39 NLT*

Father, how comforting it is to know that wherever we are, You are near. Never to forsake us. Never to leave nor distance Yourself from us. No matter what our location or our trial, You are there, nearer than our breath. Amen.

Reflection:

Reunion

The family room at the Hospice Unit was full that morning. Two women gathered at the coffee pot, chattering away. I introduced myself and my purpose in being there. They responded with an invitation to pray for their mother. Grace was now in a comatose state, but we all knew she could more than likely hear the prayer. Sweet mama was soon to meet her Lord, so I prayed for peace to fill the room and also as the sisters had wanted. "Give Mama a sweet Homecoming, Lord."

When I would return to the unit as a chaplain, I seldom met the same patients and their families. However, this second visit, five days later, did surprisingly offer me another visit with the sisters. They asked if I would officiate Mama's service since she was not from this area. I gladly accepted as long as my pastoral duties would permit at the time Mama went Home.

Service plans were made three days later. Having learned her first name was Grace, I prepared a message about the subject of God's grace. As I did, I felt an unusually strong unction to emphasize her name.

The chapel seats were filled with relatives and friends were lining the walls. I felt a release of boldness that determined itself to carry this message to God's targeted ones. Yet all I had known of this family was Grace's name and two prayer-loving sisters. Once the service was over, I witnessed the expressive warmth and love among those gathered.

How could I have known that this warm reception was unusual for this particular family? One of the sisters approached me and said, "You must learn how important this message was for our whole family!" My curiosity was raised. She continued, "My sister and I had not spoken for seven years until Mama was sick in Hospice. You see, her husband had molested my daughter, and we have been estranged ever since. He is here today, having repented for his violation, and is being loved by our family—for the first time. I forgave him and now want him back in the lives of my family members."

As I rehearsed the message the Lord had given me, I realized that I had emphasized strongly that each family member had an inheritance—an inheritance of grace. She had left deposits of grace in each one, and they were now to walk it out! All of these words flowed out of me while I was oblivious to its impact. After the family returned to their respective, out-of-state homes, I received emails stating that they were all enjoying being reunited. Grace's absence had set the stage for their absences to be filled. Only God could orchestrate such a reunion.

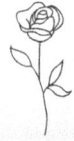 And God is able to make all grace abound to you, so that in all things at all times, having all that you need, you will abound in every good work.
—*2 Corinthians 9:8 NKJV*

Father, I am so grateful that Your prompting can touch hearts and bring reconciliation to a family. I rejoice over Your intervention in their broken relationships. May You do so in any of our relationships that beg repair. Amen.

Reflection:

The Towel

Shock would not begin to describe my reaction to the news. The call came while I was in a store–for what? I had forgotten my errand after hearing the news of our church member's sudden passing. Disbelief may have described my emotions as I wrestled with the news of my friend of 40 years. The family and I gathered at the home, trying to make sense of what had happened. Yet our sweet one was with Jesus, without a moment's notice. Laundry had just been freshly hung to dry; preceded by a two-hour phone call to another church member.

Honored to be asked to officiate her service, I knew the word to describe her life: servanthood. If her name was mentioned, most everyone would say: "She was always washing dishes or setting a table. Anything to help out." I awakened the following morning, still bewildered that this dear one was no longer with us. Then I heard these words from Holy Spirit: "Buy dish towels." "How many?" I asked Him. No reply came, which meant I was to simply obey. I purchased 30, all that was available in one style.

The funeral home chapel held 200 people and every chair was filled. Having had the Spirit's lead about towels, I focused on one of Jesus' last demonstrations of servanthood: taking up the towel of humility. "Now Jesus was fully aware that the Father had placed all things under His control, for He had come from God and was about to go back to be with Him. So He got up from the meal, took off His outer clothing, and wrapped a towel around His waist. Then He poured water into a basin and began to wash the disciples' dirty feet and dry them with His towel." (John 13:4-5)

At a time when Jesus could have been justified in thinking about the Cross before Him, instead He washed the feet of His disciples. Not only were the disciples moved by what He did, Judas saw the absence of any hypocrisy or pretense by Jesus' taking this lowly position. Servanthood is worthy of admiration. It leaves a lasting impression.

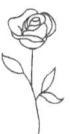
> Since God chose you to be the holy people he loves, you must clothe yourselves with tenderhearted mercy, kindness, humility, gentleness, and patience.
> —Colossians 3:12 TPT

Father, Your Son taught us that 'the way up in the Kingdom of God is down'–that is, downward into a walk of humility. This is opposite to the way our flesh would respond. Teach us Your ways of humbling ourselves and serving You and others before ourselves. And may we be ready when our time comes. Amen.

Reflection: _____

_____
_____
_____
_____
_____
_____
_____

Confession

The Hospice nurses at the local hospital guided me to the most needy patient. Their concern was that the man across the hall from their station was too stubborn to let his daughter know whether or not he was ready to meet his Maker. The nurses witnessed her sitting in the window seat, head hanging down, and anguishing over the question of her father's salvation.

Knowing I would not see him again on this side of heaven, I boldly entered the room. I found a man struggling to take some of his last breaths. His being alert enough to agree to prayer, I took his hand in mine. "Sir, I just want to make sure that we are talking to the same God. I am praying in the name of Jesus. Do you know Him?"

With his last ounce of pride, he sputtered through expiring breaths: "When you are in a fox hole in war times, and bullets are flying by your head, you make certain that you know the One who is keeping you safe!"

Having just made the most important confession of his life, he brought great relief to his daughter. Those few moments in this man's room resolved eternal business. Romans 10:9-10 clearly states that, in order to be born again, one must do two things: "If you declare with your mouth 'Jesus is Lord' and believe in your heart that God raised Him from the dead, you will be saved." Believe. Confess. This dear man had privately believed but had failed to confess with his mouth...until that day...when there was no more risk to his assurance in heaven.

As I left his room, I saw the nurses standing in line waiting to hear. With a confident hand gesture, I let them know it had been settled, both with his Lord and with his daughter. We quietly celebrated.

Paul wrote to the church at Rome that authority of Christ's resurrection was based on the scriptures:

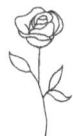 For I delivered to you as of first importance what I also received: that Christ died for our sins in accordance with the scriptures, that He was buried, that He was raised on the third day in accordance withe scriptures...
—I Corinthians 15:3-4 ESV

Father, I can sense Your presence. I have confessed that You are my Savior; I wish to make You Lord of all. You redeem all that is lost, even if it is close to our last breath. I give You praise for purchasing my salvation through Your Son Jesus. Amen.

Reflection: _____

The Whistle

Four little musical notes formed Daddy's whistle. As a little girl, I would hear him whistle those sweet sounds letting me know he was approaching. Whether he was returning from getting refreshments while we sat by the seashore, or whether he was letting me know he was home from work, Daddy's whistle thrilled me–he was here! I would exclaim: "Daddy! Daddy!"

As I grew up, Daddy didn't use that whistle anymore. Perhaps he felt it would embarrass me. He had other ways of proving his devotion. Either way, I was comforted by his presence. I was blessed to have a father who demonstrated his love for me so that I never questioned his absence. Whistle, or no whistle, Daddy was loving and faithful.

For 56 years, I treasured the demonstrations of my Daddy's love. It was when he was approaching his 91st birthday that his health was declining. I attended to his care as best I could while also caring for my ailing mother and mother-in-law. The last five days of his life were spent in the hospital, and I never left his side. At this point, Mom and my mother-in-law had passed just a few weeks before, so Daddy was my sole priority.

Sitting by his bed, I held tight, memorizing every feature of his face and hands. His vital signs were evidence that his body was on fast decline, so I assured him I was not going to leave him. I have to believe he heard every word as I thanked him for loving me so devotedly.

About 10 PM that Friday evening, somewhere in the depths of my soul, I heard the sound of my Daddy's whistle. I had not heard it for decades, so I thought it was strange that it would be resonating at this time. Two hours passed, and I heard that whistle sound again. This time I perked up, acknowledging to the Lord that I was listening. It was a couple of hours later that I heard it for the last time, very clearly. Then Daddy took his last breath on earth.

Soon after Daddy's Home going, I rehearsed the childhood whistle, realizing Daddy was letting me know he would soon be with me in our anticipated reunion in Heaven. Since he was departing from me, 56 years of memories would serve in shaping my identity and influencing my sense of well-being. This particular recollection creates a narrative that fosters Daddy's love for me, and it will last for a lifetime.

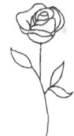

Blessed are they that mourn, for they will be comforted.
—Matthew 5:4 KJV

Father, You meet our every need. You reach into the depths of our souls and move outside of limited time to show us the magnitude of Your love. How grateful we are to You. Amen

Reflection:

The Room

Mama had just passed at 4:43 AM with Nurse Mae reading the Bible to her. Mae had witnessed my vigil at the Hospice Unit, knowing my desire to be with Mom when her time came to go Home. Being aware of my much-needed sleep, and knowing Mom's absence was near, Mae gave her the best comfort she could: God's Word.

This room had become a bit of a 'home-away-from-home' for Mom since she had spent an unusual length of time in the unit, that of 40 days. Since the average length of time in the unit was said to be 7-10 days, this extended time offered friendship and prayer time between myself and all the nurses. A gift I still enjoy, years later.

Daddy was still with us at Mom's passing, so he insisted that my husband and I take a much-needed break at our friend's bed and breakfast–at least for that one night. As soon as we left our mini-vacation site, we returned to the Hospice Unit. Mom had left her earthly home, but those I had been ministering to were still with us. My husband agreed with my need to be there and accompanied me to the nurses' station.

I asked my usual question: "Where am I needed most?" One particular patient was on their minds yet they warned me: 'there's a detail you might want to consider.' The man needing ministry had just been moved into the room my mom had occupied the entire 40 days. Their concern was that it would be too difficult for me to re-enter that very familiar room where I had spent countless hours. My reply was: "Let's go redeem the room!"

If my mom was going to be gone from my sight, leaving a great absence, I determined that another family should receive ministry, especially if it was in the same room. The reception from this loving family surrounding their alert relative was warm. Hope was released as we united in prayer, and I felt my own sense of relief. I was able to share with this dear family about my mom's faith and that she had been assured of her new home in Heaven. The patient in the same bed where Mom had declined, received prayer with his loved ones surrounding his bed. After just those few moments together, we watched him take his last breath as his face gleamed with God's peace and comfort.

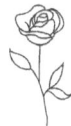 Blessed are the gentle, for they shall inherit the earth.
—Matthew 5:5

Father, only You can give us strength to move into places that otherwise could have been difficult. Your presence takes that which we have committed to You and You work in ways beyond what we could expect. We give You praise. Amen

---

Reflection:

Homestead

The front porch swing gently rocked as the breezes blew across the port city landscape As it creaked for its passenger to come have another talk, one had to wonder what it would say if the swing could talk. Well over 100 years of family life had bustled through this homestead. Generations were welcomed by its first residents and continued until the last one's passing.

Papa Dear and Mama Dear, nicknamed by my husband, were the first to set up housekeeping, raising nine children in the homestead. With hearts as big as all outdoors, they greeted family and friends. Papa Dear read the Bible to his children at night; Mama Dear had a cool glass of lemonade ready for the postman. Two rocking chairs in her bedroom were positioned for after school times with my husband. Captivated by the stories of her life, he rode his bicycle there every day after school. The house on Jefferson Street unclasped its front door like wide-opened arms as love pulsated throughout.

Take a stroll down the central hallway, from the front to the back door, you could visit what the family called 'the hall of fame.' Pictures were added as the family expanded. Years would pass and loved ones began to age and pass on. Fewer talks were heard on the front porch swing. Smiling faces still captured in the pictures in the hallway of those who went before us introduced successive generations to the faces of their honored heritage.

If the mall kitchen table for four could tattle, one would learn even more stories. Laughter filled the kitchen all hours of the day as the loved ones huddled together for small talk and a few secrets. There were times when many tears fell on the wooden table top as unwelcome changes came. The homestead was not as it once was, and hearts begged for the time clock to halt.

Established homesteads seem less prevalent these days. Young ones grow up and move away, threatening to break the links of the precious family chain. Inanimate objects cannot talk of the house on Jefferson Street, but the love that was shared for over 100 years in this homestead left indelible impressions. Memories shared within those walls, the hand waves offered until cars were out of sight, are beyond count. The bonds of love keeping families together are to be treasured, yet fewer swings rock on front porches these days. Driveways reveal lesser tire marks as generations grow up and away. As the liveliness of the hustle stills, the voices become fewer–then, silent. Longings for what was experienced in a homestead will always be a deep desire within all those who have need to belong. To capture such memories, and to hold them tight, the bonds of family ties must be preserved.

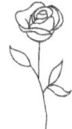 God sets the lonely in families, He leads out the prisoners with singing; but the rebellious live in a sun-scorched land. —*Psalm 68:6*

Father, the face of family is changing as we have lost some of the honor for what You have designed. Within our personal grasp, however, is the ability to preserve the ties that bind. Show us how to be the answer to this need within us all to be bonded in love. Awaken us to the need of those whom You have given us to care for; then show us how to love. Amen

Reflection:

Bargains

Having sold nearly all of their belongings in order to have better job opportunities, the young couple's hopes were high. They anticipated the upcoming school year for their three young boys. Furniture could wait; mattresses on the floor would do for now. They had each other—until the call came. We soon learned the young husband had suddenly passed away after a heart attack while at his second week of work. Having just met this family at church, I realized they braved this move with little provisions and no insurance. I spread the word among some church folks, asking for donations to help get these little boys set up for school. Gathering the sizes of the mom and children, I made my way to my favorite pennyworth store. Grabbing the checkbook, I noticed a slip of paper my husband attached: "Payday in two days. Hold off on writing checks."

Caught between following the leading of my husband and the passion to help this family, I counted the eight dollars in my wallet. Driving nearby my favorite bargain store, I felt a strong urge to go in. I reasoned I could use the layaway plan until our church folks pitched in. End of summer sales racks lined the store. $1, $3, $5 items filled my large cart to the top. After about two hours of joy-filled shopping, I approached the layaway counter and completed the information form. Two young clerks handled my items. Smiling from ear to ear, I heard one clerk say: "I'm sorry, Ma'am, but you cannot put sale items on layaway." I pled details of my story. Neither of the two women had the authority to by-pass the rules. Feeling compassion for my plight, however, they offered to re-hang all the items back on the racks. I left the store with tears welled up in my eyes. "Lord, did I miss You? I thought You instructed me to turn in to this store. These bargains!"

Upon my return home, I discovered a message on our answer machine from one of the two clerks: "Ma'am, the two of us have purchased these clothing items for you. You can pick them up when you have collected your donations, no matter how many days it takes. We have your items for you." Collections came in: just over $70. Filled with joy, I hurried to the store. The amount I owed was $52–a surprising amount as I had calculated my selections to be more. The young girls, smiling broadly, said, "We used our employee's discount." Leaving with two large bags of brand new clothing items for the children, I planned a purchase for the mom. I drove to another store, praying for yet another bargain. Just inside the door was a rack of dresses. My selection was a white, embroidered summer dress—the price? What was left over, to the dollar. No words can describe how thrilled these children were. "Mama, look what Jesus got for us!" After she wept, she opened her bag. She gasped as she pulled out the very dress that her husband had admired and promised to buy for her with his first paycheck. She wore it to his funeral.

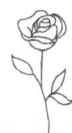 Whoever is generous to the poor lends to the Lord, and He will repay him for his deed. —*Proverbs 19:17 ESV*

Father, in times like these, we realize Your tender mercies, which are new every morning. Great is Your faithfulness. You hear our cries, and You meet the deepest desires, even the unspoken ones tucked inside a broken heart. Amen

Reflection:

Parting

Mama went back to work when I was just over two years of age. Dorothy entered my life as the one my parents trusted to care for me. Not once did she fail me. "Dottie," I nicknamed her, wrapped her plump black arms around my heart and soul and made me feel safe and secure. For eight years, she worked for our family. One of my fondest memories is that she indulged me with homemade fries–my favorite food. Never did she once complain, even if I wanted them every day. She'd peel those potatoes and fry them in the black iron skillet–just like I like them. We both enjoyed our times outside. Dottie would watch me as I learned to swing and to ride my new tricycle. She would watch as I greeted neighbors passing by. Like a sentry, she made sure I was safe and happy.

The day came when Dottie needed more salary than my parents could offer. An opportunity arose whereby she could double her income, a financial need to help put her two boys through college. The adults seemed to understand how important this was; but, to my young mind, Dottie's absence was heart-wrenching.

Both Mom and I rode the city bus to my school and to take her downtown to work for the Revenue Department. After school let out, I would ride the bus back home without mom with me. This time I would enter the house alone, without my Dottie waiting. Mama said I was old enough to be home alone until Daddy returned from work–always a bit earlier than Mom. Still, the house had an eerie quiet about it. I missed the fun times my dearest friend and I had enjoyed. Now the silence had become deafening.

I hopped on the city bus one afternoon after school and deposited my bus token in the box. Just as I turned to look for a seat, I saw my Dottie seated on the back row of the bus–right in the middle where I could see her full form. My books dropped out of my hands as I ran what seemed like a mile-long aisle to jump right into my Dottie's arms. I didn't care what anyone around her thought; in fact, I don't even remember looking into any of their faces. The only one I wanted to see was nuzzled close to my heart, saying, "Hi, Baby. I have missed you so much!" I drank from her love as much as I could, knowing the bus driver would pressure me to be seated. That was the only time I saw Dottie after she stopped working for us. Had I known this was the last time I would see her, I am sure I would have disobeyed the bus driver. This was my Dottie, and I needed her to fill that huge void in my soul.

Young children seldom understand the decisions their parents make. Whether adults are right or wrong in hat they decide to do, young minds often find it difficult to grasp. Dottie had been entrusted with my care; now she was gone out of my life. That's all I knew, and it broke my heart. There's a lasting impression left on my heart by this loving woman who served us and poured out a love that has lasted me a lifetime. These are some of the keepsakes of my soul. I can only imagine that she is in heaven among the great could of witnesses, proudly proclaiming, "That's my baby! And one day soon we will never part again!"

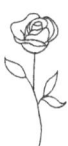 The Lord is close to the brokenhearted and saves those who are crushed in spirit. —*Psalm 34:18*

Father, I am so grateful to You for sending me such a loving caretaker and that she has her great reward in being with You. Amen.

Reflection:

Joined

Singlehood can seem very odd to one who had never lived alone. After living with college roommates, then living back at home until marriage, my times of being alone were sad. Add to that, being an only child, I promised myself that, if God graced me, I would one day have a big family to assure that I would never be alone again.

We do not have total control over how life unfolds. Our choices are strong determiners; yet, disappointment and losses come that we did not choose. I have purposed to surround myself with family and friends whom I trust to love me whether they live with me or relate from a distance. Adapting to the absences of those who have passed from this life, or those who have grown up and now build their own lives, my experiencing aloneness would never be comfortable to me.

Weeks passed after my husband's Home going before I could eat alone in a restaurant. On this singular occasion, my schedule required a meal out–alone–just before I had a pastoral counseling session. As I sat by myself in the booth, I sensed a nearness of the Lord's presence. Then I heard these words softly spoken to me: "May I join you?" His words reached my deepest need as I felt He understood. So my invisible, yet very powerfully-present Lord sat across from me in what would have been a vacant booth. He was 'being with,' a term I had come to treasure.

This encounter was the first of many to come whereby He would prove to me that He could and would be so near to my broken heart. This empty space left by those who had once filled much of my life would begin to be filled with more of Him...my new Husband. I still missed my earthly husband, the one with 'skin on.' In fact, I always will, as I long to have him hold me, to speak wisdom into my life, to share the pastorate with me, to love our children and grandchildren. Now I would get to know my new Husband who did not have 'skin on.'

Fifty-five years of marriage to my husband comforted my soul. He was always there for me. We came to understand one another as our communication deepened. His belief in me as a woman, his partner, a mother, a grandmother, and as a pastor, built a confidence. In this new venture, however, I would need to learn that Father God as my Husband had no limits in time, space, understanding, nor in resources. His unlimited supply and His desire to be my provider assured me that my needs would never be too much for Him. Nor would my encounters with Him be few.

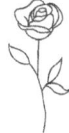

> For your Maker is your husband, the Lord of hosts is His name; and the Holy One of Israel is your Redeemer, the God of the whole earth He is called. —Isaiah 54:5 ESV

Father, I ask You: No more fears of social singleness? No more feelings of being alone? No more awkwardness among couples? You are the One with me who promised You would never leave me nor forsake me–ever! In time, I hope to rest more and more in this truth. Amen.

Reflection:

The Fog

Missing my oldest grandson's destination wedding would never have been my plan. Though the expenses were steep, nothing could keep me away from this day–or so I thought. Like a cold smack in the face, the pea-soup fog hit me. I did not want to face this beautiful occasion without my husband by my side.

Courage had shrunk up and a sense of exile had taken over. Never had I felt so excluded in social settings as I did at this time of decision. The fog swept in where once was my husband's warm companionship. Half of myself felt ripped away and my soul laid bare. I could not see a day of celebration through the denseness of this smoky view.

As I declined the invitation, another loss formed. My love for this grandson beat strong in my heart while, at the same time, I felt suddenly alone. Reasoning with myself about the joys of his union and the honor he chose by wearing his grandfather's wedding ring, I found that none of my self-talk could break through these thick vapors. He said he understood and graciously excused me; yet I knew this day would never come again. More self-talk… to no avail. Many prayers later, I just could not.

My daughter, respecting my widow's cloudy brain, sent me phone pictures and waked me through some of the wedding day details. In order to get to the wedding, she and her husband had plowed through many of the flight restrictions placed on those leaving the country. She was able to coach me through what could only be a distanced absence during this wonderful occasion.

My vulnerable moments of grief over my husband's absence swelled to include missing this grandson's beautiful beach wedding. I would learn to forgive myself as I peered through this dreaded pea-soup fog and to trust that clearer days would come again.

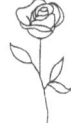 Then your light will break forth like the dawn, and your healing will quickly appear; then your righteousness will go before you, and the glory of the Lord will be your rear guard. —*Isaiah 58:8*

Father, working through the real pain of absence is no easy task. It was in those moments though that I took hold of Your presence–You being the One who understands my cloudy days and promises the sun will break through once again. Amen.

Reflection:

Shelter

Psalm 91 was his solace. Each week he would ask me to duplicate his well-worn printed copy of this psalm for him to hand out at the cancer center. I would watch him approach those waiting for their number to be called. He looked for ones who sat alone, he said. Many looked forlorn while fighting for life. We both spoke of the mournful stories that could be told by those sitting in that vast waiting room. I lost count of how many copies my husband distributed, but I do remember the faces of those who were given this beautiful psalm. After all, Psalm 91 had become a source of hope and courage to those fighting on various battlefields.

Faces lit up as the recipients realized that someone cared about their battle. Tears would stream down faces of many who shared they had gained strength from daily readings of this psalm he had given to them. Some admitted it was their first time reading it.

His gentle approach could be overheard: "I am a pastor who has found this to be very encouraging. May I give you a copy?" He was never declined. Those precious souls who crawled up under the "shadow of His wing" found the God who understands suffering in their pain-filled bodies. His shelter would be comforting and reassuring that He would never depart from them. He was the same refuge in the midst of the storm.

"He will call on Me, and I will answer him; I will be with him in trouble, I will deliver him and honor Him." —*Psalm 91:15*

Healing came to all. Some experienced it here on earth. Other, when they met their Savior on the other side. I often wonder about those who greeted my husband in heaven because of his mission to spread God's Word in that cancer center, week after bone-tiring week.

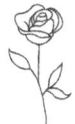 Whoever dwells in the shelter of the Most High will rest in the shadow of the Almighty. I will say of the Lord, He is my refuge and my fortress, my God, in whom I trust.
—Psalm 91:1-2

Father, Your goodness touches those who are on the battlefields of life. They are wounded warriors—battle-weary soldiers of the Living God. Your Word carries us all through times when it seems overwhelming and begging for answers. Your comfort comes, without fail, under the shelter of Your wings. Amen

---

Reflection:

Turn Right

"I have already called on this customer," he contended with the Spirit's voice. "I was just there a couple of days ago." The Voice repeated: "Turn right." The only place of business to the right was that same customer my husband had seen a few days prior. He obeyed the Lord and was greeted by the familiar receptionist. As soon as he approached her, he saw tears flowing from her eyes, along with a look of desperation.

Her husband, she explained, had left her and her young son, just days before…only after he had repeatedly abused them. Sadly, her minister had advised that she "return to her husband and submit, as the Bible said." With a confused and broken soul, she had tried to do what had been advised. Her small son, however, was found every morning hiding and sleeping under his bed after violence had stormed their home. Hope had vanished from this mother's soul so she cried out for help.

We had yet to pioneer our new church though the pastoral call had come years before. We both felt compassion for this troubled soul's cry for help, so we spent hours of counsel, giving God's hope-filled words of wisdom so that she could face her tomorrow. Jesus was her Answer.

This dear woman came to know the love of our Savior as her new life with Him began. Each step took courage as she learned how to walk with a loving Father through this uncharted path. She needed a way out; she found He IS the Way. She needed truth that would stand up under the pressures of a new walk: she learned He IS the Truth. Her life, and the life of her little son changed dramatically as she learned that He IS Life. Her walk was not promised to be an easy one, but we pledged to be by her side until she could stand strong in her new-found faith.

That still, small voice of truth can steer our pathway and bring encouragement to those who will listen. My husband's reasoning could have interfered with the plan of salvation had he failed to obey the leading of her soon-to-be-Savior.

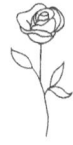

So I say, walk by the Spirit, and you will not gratify the desires of the flesh. For the flesh desires what is contrary to the Spirit, and the Spirit what is contrary to the flesh. They are in conflict with each other, so that you are not to do whatever you want. But if you are led by the Spirit, you are not under the law.
—*Galatians 5:16-18*

Father, when we yield to Your leading, fruit comes...and remains. Only You know the way that leads to the rescue of lost souls. Speak, Lord, and use us to extend a hand to those who cry out for You. May we never forget that, when we do cry out, You send help in time of need. Amen

---

Reflection:

Freedom

On certain days, when my schedule would lighten, I would ride along as my husband called on customers in nearby towns. I expected this to be a good time to read while I waited for him in the car. We were praying about planting a church, but we had not yet had the release. Soon we would learn that church is not limited to buildings.

The beautiful spring day welcomed our car windows to be opened. About halfway through the reading of my book, I felt my husband's tug at its cover. He had returned to my car in a rush and said, "I need this, right NOW!" I had learned to trust his judgment, so I gladly released it to him. Off my book went to fulfill a greater mission than I could imagine.

An appointment had been set for the secretary of this company to have shock treatments the following morning. The diagnosis by her doctor had been 'clinical depression.' hope had vanished from her soul, and despair would not let go. With my book in her hand, with my phone number written inside the cover, she would soon learn the tide was about to change.

After prayer together on the phone that first night, she cancelled her appointment. No one had told her that praise released to our Lord could open her soul's prison doors. Our new friend grabbed hold of the truth and walked into the light of God's freedom, bought just for her by Jesus Christ. Many phone calls for prayer continued. We walked with her through her journey until we were certain she could rest in this liberty. She would soon learn that praise was a weapon in her arsenal–one that would fight off the lies of the enemy.

The ones that robbed her soul of peace. It would change her pattern of thinking. It would turn her eyes heavenward to the One who could rescue her from this stormy path that she had previously walked.

Praise to Him brings focus on our God, not ourselves. The self-life can persuade us to focus on how we feel and can easily entertain the lies of doom and gloom. True hope is found only in setting our eyes on Him, where true hope is out-sourced. It chases away the enemy as it pushes back the darkness. Hissing lies will not linger in the presence of praise.

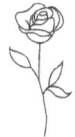 As they began to sing and praise, the Lord set ambushes against the men of Ammon and Moab and Mount Seir who were invading Judah, and they were defeated.
—2 Chronicles 20:22 KJV

Father, You inhabit the praises of Your people. Invade my soul as I lift Your name above all other names–names that would bring me down. All names must bow to the name of Jesus!. Amen!

Reflection:

The Touch

While preparing to leave for church, I answered the phone call. A friend from a town about 37 miles away called in desperate need of prayer. "I'll meet you at your church before service," she cried, "and I will explain about the liver cancer."

Our prayer team gathered around her to pray as we quietly listened to Holy Spirit to lead us. At this time, I was given a vision of my friend holding on to Jesus' robe with tenacity! Her grip was so tight, so intentional, that it seemed that, if she continued to hold on this tight, she could have been drug down the street by her grip alone. But that would not happen. She grasped hold to her only hope, Jesus. After I shared the vision with her, she left for home to spend time with the One whose robe she had grabbed.

Two days later, she reported to me that, as she had sat in her rocking chair that Sunday afternoon, weeping in God's continuing presence, she began to re-visit her past relationship with her father. Years of abandonment and pain had filled her soul. But this day would be different. She forgave him for the neglect and abuse. Just one day after prayer at church, she had returned to her oncologist's appointment. Her numbers had changed so dramatically that this puzzled doctor called for a new battery of tests.

Baffled, he reported to my friend that all cancer was GONE! No liver cancerous spots were found on the scan. She was healed!

    Did the healing touch happen when she called me on the phone that morning?

Did the healing touch happen when our team prayed together for her?

Did the healing touch happen when I shared the vision He gave me?

Did the healing touch happen as she forgave her father?

We do not know the answer to the exact time of healing manifesting and cancer cells leaving her body; however, we can celebrate the results that came directly from the Healer.

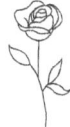 And when the woman saw that she was not hid, she came trembling, and falling down before Him, she declared unto Him before all the people for what cause she had touched Him, and how she was healed immediately. —*Luke 8:47 ESV*

Father, just one touch from Jesus is all it takes for healing to come to me. I give You my fears, my pains, my body aches, and any sickness. I trust the stripes placed on Jesus' back to absorb every one of them, in Jesus' name. Amen!

Reflection:

God Kind of Faith

Her screams roared through the phone, so much so that I had to ask the woman to please identify herself. My friend gathered herself just enough to let me know who she was and that I needed to come. Her eyesight was gone. I called a nearby church friend to come stay with my small children while I rushed to Sandy's side. Bible in hand, I knew this was the best I could give her. She had battled severe diabetes for a long time. Now the lights were out and she was frantic. As I arrived, I knew her emotional state was beyond my reasoning with her, so I opened to Psalms. And I read. She screamed and cried while I continued to read, undeterred.

Holy Spirit spoke that she was to repeat the scriptures after me. Agitated, she resisted me and said 'NO!' She was persuaded she could not do so I shook her shoulders and commanded she look at me. I said, "This you WILL do! Do you hear me? You WILL repeat after me." I must say that this was not my usual approach. A boldness that was beyond my own power had taken over—a force that was way beyond myself. I knew the word of God going forth was the only remedy to her need. It took some repeated times of reading and waiting on her before Sandy began to muffle a few of the words. Still panic-stricken, she found it very difficult to cooperate. HIS faith in me persisted. Minutes had passed before I watched Sandy's eyes begin to focus. Little by little, the word of God began to manifest her healing. I saw it happen right in front of me! Her eyes cleared up, and sight returned, very clear! We were both elated as we rejoiced and danced around the room, celebrating the power of God's word.

On my way home, I began to realize for the first time that it had never crossed my mind to take her to the doctor nor the hospital. Because God had given me HIS faith, I was able to walk out His instructions, without any doubt. His faith made it possible for me to follow His instructions, with His boldness, to accomplish what He had planned as Healer.

This was my first encounter with the gift of faith, the God-kind-of-faith, which is beyond our own measure of faith given to us. This kind of faith pole-vaults us way beyond anything we could even imagine within our own sphere of belief. It's the special gift where, by the Spirit of God, provides Christians with extraordinary confidence in His promises, power, and presence so they can take heroic stands for His work. It's unshakable confidence in Him, His word, and His promises. It's where miracles happen, as it did that day for Sandy. And her sight returned and remained. All because He provided HIS faith through a simple vessel.

Paul wrote to the Corinthians about this particular spiritual gift. He stated: *"To another faith by the same Spirit, to another the gifts of healing by the one Spirit."* **(I Corinthians 12:9 NRSV)**

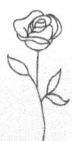 Now faith is the assurance of things hoped for, the conviction of things not seen. —*Hebrews 11:1 ESV*

Father, use me whenever You want to, in order to bless others. Your faith is powerful and it knows no hindrances. Thank You for displaying Your glory! Amen.

Reflection:

All In

During worship in the early years of pioneering our church, the Spirit of God spoke these words to me: *May I interrupt this program to have church?* Stunned, I immediately wondered what we were doing wrong, right in the midst of a powerful worship song. He added, *It's not what you are doing wrong; it's what I want to teach you to do right.* As surrendered as I could be at that time, I said that I would carefully listen to His leading, if He would give me His grace. After all, as a church, we desired His presence; not His absence.

Years later, I cannot say that we have mastered this, yet we humbly bow before Him as best we know how. His voice from that early encounter still rings profoundly in my soul. A promise was made that day that, given His grace, I would lead our flock into what He desired. He has taught us as a congregation that His presence and purpose was and is all that matters to Him; anything added to or taken away would be less than His design. That led me and my husband to a place of learning dependence on His guidance, forgetting any preconceived ideas we had about what church services should be like.

At several intersections of time, He would ask me: *What impresses you?* I understood Him to imply that whatever impressed me was what drew my attention, my affection, and therefore my actions. This inventory still causes me to stay close to hearing from the One who desires to lead me in His ways...dependent upon His grace.

One Sunday, He asked: *Are you all in?* A vision followed that reminded me of a television commercial I had seen years ago showing twin sisters being so overwhelmed by pleasure with a certain food item that they fell backwards into a swimming pool. The vision, however, was presented to me in extremely slow motion. He allowed me to imagine the twins stopping mid-air before hitting the water, deciding whether they wanted to finish the fall. I soon realized that once the plunge was taken, there was no turning back. Again, He asked: *Are you all in?*

His presence, His purpose. No more than; no less than. From Him we receive strength and hope in the tough times. We come to know Him more fully. Even when we are alone, we are not lonely.

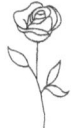 Yea, though I walk through the valley of the shadow of death, I will fear no evil; for You are with me; Your rod and Your staff, they comfort me. —*Psalm 23:4 NKJV*

Father, my desire is to take the plunge–not to stop midway. I wish to fall deeper in love with You, without indecisions slowing me down. Your invitation remains. Help me to be 'all in.' Amen

---

Reflection: _____

Full Joy

As she entered the door, she said, "Without a doubt, you cannot help me now. I have been suicidal all week, contemplating different ways to snuff out my life. I cannot take it anymore!" The prayer team invited her to a time of prayer where we could seek what the Lord would say. She agreed. Healing prayers had helped her before; but, this time, she was stuck in a rut that seemed terribly deep. We listened and heard her explain multiple answers for why she was the exception to the good news of the gospel. The Word was no longer going to work for her, she said, because she was too far gone. That is: in her estimation. We lifted her desperate cry before the Lord and listened to His instruction. He's the only One who can fix our broken places.

He brought to my spiritual eye a vision of an arcade shooting game. He instructed that I ask her to tell me the first 'reason' she was exempt from being set free. She named her reason. Then she smiled as I asked her to hold up her pretend gun and shoot it down. I asked her to name a second 'reason' she was the exception to what the Word revealed about being set free. She named the second one, and aimed her gun. As she began to list her 'reasons,' her eyes began to brighten. The lies became apparent as she spoke each one of them. She heard herself and giggled as the lies no longer made sense. With each 'reason,' she became more and more persuaded that she had been basing every though on the lies of the enemy.

"Ask, and you will receive, that your joy may be full." (John 16:24b NKJV)

By the time this dear one finished listing about six lies, and shooting each one of them down with her pretend gun, she accepted her God-given freedom. Her giggles became hilarious laughter. So much joy filled her that she went to her knees. Then to the floor...completely undone by the weight of joy overtaking her. Our prayer team celebrated with her as we helped her to her car. This woman was completely changed from the absence of hope to the powerful presence of God's personal touch on her soul.

This breakthrough for our sister remained solid for the remaining days of her life. Joy sustained her and dwelt within, despite circumstances she did not live to see change. Happiness is fleeting because it is centered on what is happening at a given time. She began to write anointed poetry and to share God's victory with her lost family members. The day of her memorial service was one of immense celebration as her family rejoiced that this one had found lasting freedom–freedom from a very dark place that could have brought very serious results.

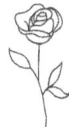 A joyful heart is good medicine, but a crushed spirit dries up the bones. —*Proverbs 17:22 ESV*

Father, no matter how dark the valley, You are deeper still. There's no place we can hide from or run to that You are not waiting to rescue us. Show me the way out of my dark places today, Lord. I long for Your light and glory. Amen.

Reflection: _____

This Way

The young man was at a decision crossroad. He listed several positive reasons for the first decision; then he listed some of the negatives. Frustrated, he continued to argue about his rights to make these decisions on his own. After all, he declared, "I am of age!"

In a tenuous place as his counselor, I could have caused more confusion by inserting my own opinions. A silent prayer went heavenward: "Lord, I ask that You give me Your wisdom. Help me to assist this young man to see clearly and, in turn, for him to choose to listen to You."

The answer came. "Ask him this question: Would you rather have a map or a Guide?" I posed the question and waited. His reply was: "Can I have both?" I had to laugh out loud because I could relate to the temptations in 'mapping out' my own life. My answer to him was that I believed the Lord's wisdom required the choosing of one OR the other.

We spent a little time discussing how 'mapping out' our own desires can not only lead us astray, but can delay the fulfilling of our destiny. Detours can always lead back to the main road; however, who wants to design a journey of detours? These detours only delay God's ultimate plan and often require a great deal of clean up.

Next, we discussed the wisdom of walking with the Guide: Holy Spirit. His directions are always clear, and they lead us onto straight paths.

"Trust in the Lord with all your heart, and lean not unto your own understanding. In all your ways acknowledge Him, and He will make your paths straight." (Proverbs 3:5-6)

This young man welcomed the word from the Lord and even shared this truth with many of his friends. Did he walk with the Guide or choose his own mapping? The answer to this question is not mine to judge. I was only to deliver the question. My guess is that he will learn to choose both, never forgetting any consequences.

Delays and detours have certainly peppered my life. They can and do turn out to be life lessons, if we learn from them. However, the walk is sweeter and more certain when we trust the Guide and obey His leading.

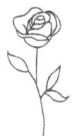 Your ears shall hear a word behind you, saying, This is the way, walk in it, whenever you turn to the right hand or whenever you turn to the left. —*Isaiah 30:21*

Father, I need Your guidance, not my own leading. Prone to wander, I can easily map out my own way of planning and find myself on the proverbial side roads of life. Help me to hear Your voice, and to heed Your will. Amen

Reflection:

Mighty Mite

As a young child, one of our granddaughters collected all the monies she had and counted it carefully. Christmas was coming, and she wanted to give something to each of her family members. Calling me on the phone, she asked the exact number of those who planned to attend our big holiday reunion. Then she divided the sum of her money by that number.

The value on a gift is relative. To this child's mind, all of the money she had earned doing little chores for us was quite valuable to her. So to divide it into smaller amounts still displayed the overflow of a generous heart.

Years have passed now, yet this is a memory none of those present will forget. Paper and ribbons tossed from one corner of the room to the other as excitement arose that Christmas holiday. Big and smaller packages were opened with many expressions of gratitude. Then my granddaughter pulled from her backpack a zipped bag for each person there. Inside the bag was 27 cents she had counted out equally. It is impossible to express the impact these gifts made on the hearts of those receiving them. The 'mighty mite' made a loud impression. An older grandson later confessed to tears welling up in his eyes when she gave offered her gifts.

On another holiday occasion, our youngest granddaughter saved her birthday money and chore earnings to shop at the dollar store. Careful selections were made as she remembered the special interests of each person. Purchases made, gifts wrapped, it was evident that the highlight of her holiday was not in receiving of gifts but in giving something selected with love for her family.

Jesus put enormous value on the widow's mite. "Truly I say to you that this poor widow has put in more than all; for all these out of their abundance have put in offerings for God, but she out of her poverty put in all the livelihood that she had." (Luke 21:3-4 NKJV) The widow's two mites, Roman coins called 'lepton,' were worth the value of six minutes' of average daily wages. In Western measure of money, this is worth about a penny. It is easy for us to overlook the smaller gifts, but Jesus saw the humble gift of the widow. Though the rich were giving large sums, they still retained their fortunes. The widow put in everything she had–a true sacrifice. In need of charity for herself, she had a heart to give. Her 'mighty mite' impressed our Lord.

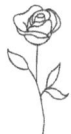

...But out of her poverty put in all the livelihood that she had. —*Luke 21:4*

Father, You value the loving intentions of our heart. Help us to remember that even the smallest of sacrificial gifts are seen by You and valued by others. Open our hearts to release even that which costs us our all. Amen.

Reflection:

The Squeeze

Our teachers can be some of the greatest influences in our lives–hopefully for the good. Those who have had the greatest impact on my life have been some of the ones who were tough on me. Driving out the tendency to slack, to take 'the easy way out,' was not a simple task for school teachers nor mentors.

The day came when I learned that I had been placed in an advanced English class with Phyllis Peacock. Her reputation preceded her; from her classes came prepared college material. Many of her students would become authors as well as achieve professional careers. How I came to be placed in her class puzzled me; in fact, it scared me. Intimidated, my first 9 weeks' reporting period reflected the absence of discipline. Yet I'll never forget her pulling me out of one of my classes, pleading with me to understand that she had averaged my grades more than once, only to find that I was due to receive an "F" on my first report card. Her sincerity was so evident that I found myself reassuring her! When the report card came, she had given me a "D."

That gifted letter propelled me forward. I was more determined than ever to work harder to receive her favor. Upon giving her class requirements even more attention, it caused my other teachers to compete. One department was offering me a scholarship, and the teachers were vying for more of my extra curricula time. Not only did I work harder to understand what Mrs. Peacock was needing from me, I was given opportunity to earn extra credit by teaching my class three new vocabulary words every day. The next report card reflected my efforts, and I was happy to say that by the third reporting period, I had achieved "A's." She became my favorite teacher. In my twenties, I re-dedicated my walk with the Lord and realized my need for mentoring. Having several women in church who had walked with the Lord more years than myself, I submitted myself to their teachings. One in particular took the time to walk with me day by day. My goal was to do the things she suggested: study the Word, practice godly attitudes, and allow her to train me. Then I would check in with her for my spiritual 'report card.' I longed for her approval, so I bragged on how diligent I had been in fulfilling her suggested assignments. Then, as usual, I would hear the dreaded words: "My dear..." When those words came, I white-knuckled myself for the truth that sets you free–but first, it sure can squeeze the soft places of the flesh–those places where there is definite absence of discipline. Decades later, I am still quoting my intimidating teacher and my mentor. Wisdom flowed from them, though most of the time their demands were tough.

Both of them drove truth into my soul that could not wiggle its way out. Bragging on my efforts, and trying to impress, I would hear my mentor say: "My dear, it is not YOURS until you flesh it out!" Over and over again, my lame efforts to receive stamps of approval from these who invested in me did not deter them from discipline. At the same time, they never gave up on me. Their personally disciplined lives qualified them to discipline mine.

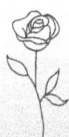 For the moment all discipline seems painful rather than pleasant, but later it yields the peaceful fruit of righteousness to those who have been trained by it.
—Hebrews 12:11

Father, I can see that my life has been greatly affected by those You sent to bring shape and form to my life. I welcome Your ways that bring transformation to my soul. Amen.

Reflection: _____

_____
_____
_____
_____
_____
_____
_____
_____
_____
_____
_____
_____
_____

Lost But Found

Unpacking from travels, I realized my plastic, wide-tooth comb was missing. I admit it had been helpful when combing my wet hair yet I reasoned the dollar item was an easy replacement. Still curious, I asked my husband if he had seen it. I had looked through both suitcases, checked the bathroom counter more than once, looked in the car, and even searched places I knew it could not have been. He joined me in the search, but to no avail.

Rehearsing in our minds that the comb was cheaply replaced, we were still impressed to continue our search. My last effort was to look on the bathroom counter, where the comb usually laid. There it was–right in plain sight–on my counter. There was no way that he and I could have missed the obvious. No doubt to either of us, an angel had returned my comb to me. Dollar's worth or not, the angel let me know that even the smallest of things that concern me matter to Father God.

My oldest daughter had been given an add-a-pearl necklace by her godparents. Each birthday, a new pearl would join the others and lengthen the chain. Dressing for our Sunday night church service, she decided to wear one of her favorites, which she persuaded us needed the necklace to make her happy. After service, she and the other children ran the church yard, jumping up and down with joy. As we were leaving, she noticed her necklace was missing. Equally noticeable was the 6" height of the grass, which was to be mowed the following day. Finding that necklace in the midst of tall grass seemed an impossibility. Church friends stopped what they were doing and helped us in the search.

Not five minutes passed and my daughter squealed, "I've found it!" The necklace was laying in a little cluster, hiding in 6"-tall grass. Unbroken and still in tact, the necklace must have slipped over her head while she romped during this time of playfulness. Once again Father God let us know He cares about every detail.

Both husband and son enjoyed sneaking an ice cream treat, especially without my knowing it. They anticipated I would speak to their consciences about the undesirable calories. They pulled in the driveway and raced to the trash can to hide the evidence and its cup holder. The following morning, my son was very upset that his wallet had once again gone missing. Inside was money he had earned working many hours for a friend's father. I urged him to cool his emotions and to ask the Lord where he put it. When he finally settled down to pray, he received the Lord's prompting. He hurried out the door and opened the lid to the trash can. There, among the evidence was his wallet, laying underneath the cup holder. Adding emphasis to this valued discovery was the fact that it was 'trash day.' In less than an hour, the cans would have been on the street, with evidence and wallet being forever lost.

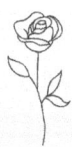

The Lord directs the steps of the godly. He delights in every detail of their lives. —*Psalm 37:23 NLT*

Father, there's nowhere we can go, nor are there things that concern us, out of Your sight. You know all things, and You make them known to us as we have need. Your presence is precious in every step of our journey. Amen.

Reflection:

Pop Quizzes

Two local teams had been rivals for several years, so emotions mounted as the score became uncomfortably close. Parents walked the sides of the field and yelled some encouraging words; some yelling words not repeatable. Coach wiped his sweaty, red face as his blood pressure was obviously mounting. Tensions were high throughout the stadium.

Game over—and our team had lost to its biggest rival. Coach was furious, as he had seen game plays for the past hour that did not meet his instructions. So he commanded the team off the field and into the field house. In prior games, however, he had taught them about sportsmanship. Shake hands, even if you have suffered an embarrassing loss to your opponent. Fury caused him to react differently this homecoming game of the season. The loss was too much for him to handle.

Confused, our team players remembered this was not the way they had behaved in prior games–winning or losing. Yet Coach had yelled the command. One young team player weighed out a decision: would he risk being kicked off the team, if he did what he felt was the right thing to do?

The risk was taken. He left the field house. To his great surprise, the opposing team members had already been lined up by their coach, waiting for our team players to emerge from the field house. This young man was the only one who did. He walked the length of the line and shook hands with each of the winning players. Our son's character spoke for itself.

Grandfather had emphasized to this young boy that anyone who had served in the Armed Forces was always to be honored. They serve our country and are due our respect, he taught him. This six-year-old young boy remembered his wisdom at breakfast one morning. His grandfather had set their food down at the selected booth and then went to pour his coffee. As he returned to the booth, the boy was missing.

He looked all over the room and found the young boy sitting in a booth with a man whose ball cap logo announced him to be a veteran. After a few words and a handshake, the boy returned to grandfather's booth and explained that he had remembered to thank those who were presently serving or had served in the military, so he was doing just that. Reprimands were withheld, as our grandson's character was speaking for itself. Life is full of 'pop quiz' encounters. God allows them as character tests. We do not pass them all. Some we fail miserably. He is, however, gracious enough to give us more opportunities to do what is right. May we not forget that His mercies even curve our grade.

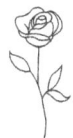 You shall do what is right and good in the sight of the Lord, that it may be well with you, and that you may go in and possess the good land which the Lord swore to give your fathers. —*Deuteronomy 6:18*

Father, I'm aware that life is full of 'pop quiz' encounters. It appears that You allow them as true character reveals. We do not pass all these tests; some we fail miserably. You prove, however, to be gracious in giving us more opportunities to do what is right. As for our final grading period, we are assured that Your mercy and grace have curved our grade. Amen!

Reflection:

Onlies

He made me feel like I was the only one in the room. Daddy would introduce me to his friends as his 'favorite child.' As I would hear those words each time, I noticed his words stirred up my feelings of discomfort. What bothered me was that Daddy was saying something that I felt was untrue; and my daddy was too amazing in my eyes to do anything less than perfect.

I am an only child. In my way of thinking, Daddy was telling a lie. Maybe I did not call it an actual lie: as that word seemed far too harsh. Still, in my mind, his introduction was exaggerated, causing people to think I was one of multiple children. I would wring and twist in place, then look into Daddy's face begging, "Dad-eeeee!" I wanted him to explain to his friends that he was not telling the truth, and that I was his one and only child. I needed him to make it right.

I struggled with this 'favorite child' introduction until I was in my 20's. Three years into marriage, we began having our children—one after another—until we had three children ages four and under. It was at this point in time that I crumbled under the weight of responsibility and cried out to the Lord for His strength, His wisdom, and for Him to be more than just my Savior: to be my Lord. As my walk began to mature, I realized how easy it was for me to believe I was loved by Father God. In fact, I grew to feel that I was HIS only child. Though I knew others enjoyed that closeness too, what remained most important to me was that I was His and He was mine. We were 'onlies.'

What a set up! Daddy's teases meant he sincerely loved me. But that set up prepared me to believe also in Father's love. Just as God has designed it, our parents are the first demonstration of Father's love to us as children. Daddy had done it so well. He set me up to believe and to receive Father God's love.

At school, children would tease me about being an 'only,' and I struggled with that label because it felt like something was wrong with me. Only later did I realize that Daddy had set me up for one of the greatest revelations I could ever have in my walk with God. He and I are 'onlies.' What's more: all of His children are to experience being His 'onlies.'

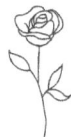 Just as the Father has loved Me, I have also loved you; abide in My love. —*John 15:9*

Father, there's nothing more satisfying than feeling safe in Your love and shepherding care. You never fail to reveal how much You love us. If only we paid attention to Your repeated expressions throughout our days. Open our hearts to know You more and to feel this love You pour upon us. Amen.

Reflection:

Marked

What seemed like a trip to the bank became much more. In my personal way of acknowledging Holy Spirit's promised presence with me, I will often extend my hand to the passenger side of my car. It's my way of letting Him know that I know He's with me and I am grateful. As I extended my hand of welcome this day, I began to experience His presence—not simply by faith. The power of His Spirit filled my car and caused me to begin to cry all the way to the bank. I'm not sure what the teller at the window thought of me, but it did not matter. I had Him.

After the banking transition, I extended my hand once again to my car's passenger side. This time, I felt His fingers touch each one of the fingers on my right hand—matching fingertips to fingertips. This was far more than I could have imagined or even asked for. My thoughts immediately went to frequent questions I had been asked about my pastoral views of tattooing one's body. To avoid implying condemnation, I would hold up my thumb and call attention to the fact that I have my own tattoo, one with which the Lord has marked my body. I added: "There is not another one in the world like it. And you have one too!"

When I arrived back home, I went online to read about the divine formation of our fingerprints in the womb. I learned that it was during the early weeks that our little finger pads were formed, but, in the last trimester, the prints were etched upon those miniature pads. "When I consider the heavens, the work of Thy fingers…" (Psalm 8:3)

Father God has left His signature upon each one of us, lest we ever forget how precious we are to Him. Ephesians 1:4: "For He chose us in Him before the creation of the world to be holy and blameless in His sight in love."

Further study on fingerprint led me online to an artist who enlarged a picture of a fingerprint after reading about the fingerprint of God. As he studied the print, he realized that each one has 66 lines etched upon it. He hand-wrote a scripture from each of the 66 books in the Bible upon each tiny line. That art work was made available; therefore my copy hangs matted and framed on our church wall.

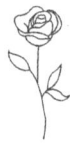

> ...Even there Your hand will guide me, Your right hand will hold me fast...."I praise You because I am fearfully and wonderfully made, Your works are wonderful, I know that full well. My frame was not hidden from You when I was made in the secret place, when I was woven together in the depths of the earth. Your eyes saw my unformed body; all the days ordained for me were written in Your book before one of them came to be.
>
> —*Psalm 139:10; 14-16*

Father, as I walk with You, may I never forget that I am marked by You. Your signature has established Your love for me and how You value Your creation. Before the sun, moon and stars were formed, You were planning my life. How precious each of Your children are in Your sight. Amen.

Reflection:

Retreat

Early mornings with my Lord are treasured times set aside to give Him the first fruits. Never do I leave with only what I have given to Him. In this particular encounter, He called for a retreat—a time that was open-ended until we dealt with what was on His mind. His instruction was: "Before going up to the high places, I am going to heal the hurts of your past." Faces and names that came to my mind were those whom I had already purposed to forgive. What was to be addressed once and for all were the wounds left in my soul.

The 'higher places' mentioned in Ephesians 6:12 reference spiritual wickedness in high places. "For we wrestle not against flesh and blood, but against principalities, against powers, against the rulers of the darkness of this world, against spiritual wickedness in high places." His instruction to me was that, if I am to progress in Kingdom of God ministry, I will need to be free of any stumbling blocks that would hinder me.

This early morning time with Him became a two-day retreat that He ordained. One by one, each hurt was addressed. I acknowledged what He called to my mind, told Him how much it hurt, and then released the stored-up pain to Him. Some of these hurts had remained so tucked within that I had become accustomed to carrying them. Relationships that I found to be challenging had become a part of me. The residue of their hurtful impact had left familiar bruises in my soul. He wanted them all, and I love Him for it.

Deliverance came as each hurt broke free. I took very few breaks over these two days, as the work He was doing was effective, leaving me with a deeper revelation of His love than I had never known. His instructions were that, before I could move to the next assignment He ordained, I had to be freed from these hurts. If not, they would become the filter through which I would relate to others.

The threshold of pain surrounding each hurt prompted me to be willing to release. I had carried them way too long. My Lord cared about everything my soul had in its storehouse. Anything keeping me from going to the higher places had to be removed. I would need to be reminded that I do not fight flesh and blood—though the wounds I was submitting to Him had come directly from the enemy making it indirectly from human beings. This would need to become an established truth.

He parked me, and I did not desire to move from that divine encounter until He considered it a finished assignment. As for the wounds, I don't know 'where' they went; I am not searching them out. I do know 'how' they went—by my beloved Shepherd who restored my soul.

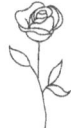 No one can come to Me unless the Father who sent Me draws him. And I will raise him up on the last day.
— *John 12:32*

Father, How grateful I am that You drew me to Yourself. The precious times together with Holy Spirit, healing my wounds, reveal how deep Your love is for me. Amen.

Reflection:

Break Through

Stained-glass windows were my first glimpse of Jesus in art form. Beautiful artisan work on three sides of my family's church walls invited me into a reality of Jesus. I do not ever remember doubting that He was real. These windows, ceilings, and panels have captivated lovers of beauty for over a thousand years. Constructed pieces that are connected and outlined by strips of lead offered my first reflection of light breaking through walls.

Jesus did not step out of the panels of colorfully etched pieces until my salvation at thirteen years of age. My wonderful Savior became more personal than crafted art. My soul began a transformational journey through which He planned His light to shine in me and through me. Though it has been many years that I have walked with Him, I remain grateful for artisans who taught me about Him through the original craft. However, He had so much more of Himself to reveal as He walked into and through the walls of my heart. "The Word became flesh," remains one of the most celebrated acts of love Father God has expressed to mankind. (John 1:14) Jesus becoming flesh—the Living God becoming the Son of Man—offered us the way out of our hopeless darkness, from behind stubborn walls. Light came through our Savior; He stepped out of and beyond the etchings of stained glass and offered to come into our hearts—as He did mine.

Father God's intentions have always been to reveal Himself as the one who is relevant to man's desperate craving for intimacy. Until He steps beyond the craftsman's admirable work and into an individual's heart that welcomes "the Word becoming flesh," He will remain a fictional story, remote and impersonal. Just colored glass through blind or distorted vision.

Jesus was not to be bound to a beautiful window, though its elegance remains pleasing to the eye. Absence from the soul of man is the travesty. He was never to remain limited to the religious boxes erected by man's intellectual pride. What has kept glorious biblical truths confined to ink on paper has suffered the absence of the life-breathing essence of the Holy Spirit. Stepping out of the pages of the Bible comes the one who became flesh and who calls us to an Eden-like experience. The Genesis account (2:4-6) reveals how He intended our walks to be. My Daddy's favorite lyrics were: "My God and I walk through the fields together. We walk and talk as good men should and do. We clasp our hands, our voices ring with laughter. My God and I walk through the meadow's hue." (My God and I, by Austris Whithold, 1971).

The actual truth about the Son of Man who was the most human of all humanity can sadly be confined to man's entrapments. Those detainments of His majesty have set limits on the fullest expression of who He really is and what He wants to make known to us about Himself. Just when we think we might know Him, He surprises us with another facet of His vast wealth of glory.

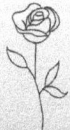 Your Son is magnificent; He can never be praised enough. —*Psalm 145:3 MSG*

Father, our concepts of You are confined by what we 'think' we know about You; yet there is so much more to know of You, beyond our self-made walls. We must set 'who You are' free from our intellectual imprisonment. Show us Your glory, Lord! Amen.

Reflection:

Glory

"Heaven came down and glory filled my soul. When at the cross the Savior made me whole. My sins were washed away, and my night became as day. Heaven came down and glory filled my soul." This song. Written by John W. Peterson (1921), erupted from memory as I prayed He would display His glory during our church service that morning.

He had prompted me to meditate on 'glory' many days prior. As I did, I struggled to comprehend what the glory actually was and is. Feeling totally inept at grasping the stunning concept of glory, I pled for understanding. He explained that holiness is His very essence. There's none with which to compare. He is in a class all His own. So holiness was described to me as the centrality of His nature, revealing who He is. Out from His holiness come the manifestations of His glory. I will refer to them as 'glory rays,' like the rays coming forth from the sun. "Heaven came down…"

"When at the cross the Savior made me whole." Glory was made available through the shed blood of Jesus Christ to whosoever would believe in Him and call upon Him to save their souls. His glory made wholeness available spirit, soul, and body. "My sins were washed away…" meant more glory was dispensed as the powerful cleansing agent. "My night became as day." Glory radiates; darkness cannot survive.

Now that "heaven has come down and glory has filled our souls," we carry the glory within our spirit man. He is in us, and we are in

Him, Paul admonished the church at Ephesus. The glory resides in His children as our "night became as day."

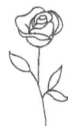 The heavens are telling the glory of God. —*Psalm 19:11*

Father, Your glory cannot be contained. The heavens and the earth display the splendor of Your majesty. In Your perfect plan to open the eyes of those who did not know You, You sent Your Son—the fullest expression of Your holiness. Love came down. Glory came down. Your glory provided us so great a salvation, and now Your glory fills those of us who have chosen You to be our Lord. Amen

Reflection:

One-on-One

In our world of easy access to the opinions and experiences of others, we can miss our Lord. Finding Him for ourselves is the key to experiencing the abundant life He came to give us. Habitual searches in learning more about my Lord are from those I admire and trust. I can easily fall into a pattern of letting them search for me, teach me, and even inspire me, instead of researching for myself.

I sat before the television set one night, Bible in hand, notepad on my knee, listening to one I trust to bring me richness from the Word of God. Attentive and excited, I was ready to receive when I heard the Spirit of God say: "I miss you." My warm response was: "That's so dear." After scribing a few more notes, I heard the same kind voice again:

> "I miss you." He had my attention, so I debated with Him that this man was bringing me such a wonderful understanding of how to walk by the Spirit. "Wait for me. This program will be over in just a few minutes." The sound of His silence became deafening.

I immediately turned off the television and headed to my quiet place of altar. I asked him to forgive me for delaying and debating over His "missing me" He began to teach me a lesson I will never forget. The teacher who was bringing forth rich revelation had received that for himself. Holy Spirit wanted to teach me about Himself—no middle person. He explained that I may read a menu about the most delicious foods being prepared; but, if I do not order and eat the meal, I am still hungry. If a person describes to me what meal they just ate, giving me details of the color, the taste, the satisfaction in their palate; I remain hungry, if I do not eat that meal. No matter how persuasive the menu, nor the testimony, I remain unsatisfied. Therefore, what was being taught by way of another's experience was inspiring, no doubt; yet it did not make direct contact with my own hunger and thirst. His desire was to feed me Himself.

There's nothing like personal revelation served by the one who is the Bread of life. The Water of life: one who stirs up rivers of living water within our soul…the one who beckons us to "taste and see that the Lord is good." In a dry and thirsty land, He invites us to "earnestly seek Him. "I thirst for You, my whole being longs for You, in a dry, and parched land where there is no water." (Psalm 63:1)

No doubt, I was dry and thirsty. That's why I was so intent upon the teaching this anointed man was offering. Yet, there was the direct access to the Teacher of all teachers, one-on-one feeding, from the one who would bring fresh manna directly into my soul.

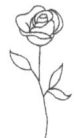 …For me it is good to be near God. —*Psalm 73:28*

Father, second-hand meals do not satisfy. Leftovers from another's table leave much to be desired. I want first-hand servings from Your table You prepare for me. May I never delay when You call me to dine. Feed my hungry soul, Lord. Amen.

Reflection:

Abba

Daily devotional greetings with my Lord begin with these words: "Abba, I belong to You." They are never empty words; they render power from the reality of *to whom I belong*. This posture sets my day in order, as I surrender myself to Him, His plan for my day, and bring to remembrance the days that I have chosen my own path which bore little to no lasting fruit.

The warmth of this reality continues throughout the day, as I reflect upon those words at intervals, pausing and thanking Him that He first chose me. "You did not choose Me, but I chose you and appointed you so that you might go and bear fruit—fruit that will last—and so that whatever you ask in My name the Father will give you." (John 15:16)

Belonging is a deep inner need of every person…the need of a very personal or private relationship. The closeness, the affections shared, the constancy of His presence remove any feelings of distance. Father God has made each of us to need this belonging—most importantly to Himself. That hunger will never be satisfied by another person, nor another thing. The absence of that belonging creates an 'orphaned' soul.

At least 100 times the Gospels record Jesus calling God 'Father.' For example, He taught His disciples to pray: "Our Father…." (Matthew 6:9) They had watched Him take time to depart from their company to spend time alone with His Father. They too wanted to belong. The only time Jesus ever called His Father anything other than 'Father' was on the Cross. Bearing the sin and shame of the world upon Himself, Jesus was 'orphaned' from His Father in those hours, and thereby twice called Him 'God.' (Matthew 23:46) How difficult it is to imagine what those hours must have been for the Holy One to be separated—for the first time—from His deepest bond. Yet He did this for me. And for you.

Whenever He referred to Father, those terms were intimate, connecting one with the other, nothing withstanding. Yet, at Calvary, that voluntary separation between Father and Son to a place of remote, relational experience, tore the veil between God and His children. Therefore, we ony need to cry, "Abba, Father."

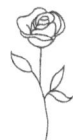

> The Spirit you received does not make you slaves, so that you live in fear again; rather, the Spirit you received brought about your adoption to sonship. And by Him we cry, 'Abba, Father.' —*Romans 8:15*

Father, Your word draws us to You. The power of Your love is strong and causes us to long for more of You. How can we ever turn away from Your invitation to be fathered by You? We cry, "Abba!" Amen.

Reflection:

Identity Theft

"Whom do you say that I am?" Jesus inquired of the disciples. How important it was to Him to be known as He truly was, and is. This question provoked an answer from those gathered around Him. Peter's response is the only one recorded. That leaves us to believe the others either had no idea, or they were stumped by the question.

He asked His disciples in private who the crowds said He was. They replied, "Some say John the Baptist; others say Elijah; and still others, that one of the prophets of long ago has come back to life. (Luke 9:20). Peter answered: "God's Messiah." (9:18-20) He was accurate—at least until he balked about Jesus leaving them—then received a terrible rebuke from the Lord. The thief was at work in his mind.

Jesus was not oblivious of their opinions of Him; He knew all things. Neither was this a question regarding vanity. He wanted to provoke their faith. "Blessed are you, Simon son of Jonah, for this was not revealed to you by flesh and blood, but by My Father in heaven." (Matthew 16:17) Suffering was forecasted for Jesus; therefore, His disciples needed to be settled in their faith. Hard times would come causing them to be thrown into confusion, if faith was absent. Asking this question demanded of them a considered response.

Religion has been the greatest thief of Jesus' true identity. He has been misrepresented from the day He was born. Prophets had recorded the coming Messiah, His sufferings, along with His divine attributes. While scribes and Pharisees knew these recorded words, they missed knowing The Word who stood right in front of them in the flesh.

Before we become judgmental of these thick-skulled intellectuals, we must realize that we too have had misconceptions of who He really is. How quickly we forget what He has done for us at Calvary. How easily we condemn ourselves and others when He made it known that we were to love Him with all our hearts, souls, minds, and strength, and our neighbor as ourselves. (Luke 10:27) Believe it or not, He even had a sense of humor and laughed!

No one likes to be misrepresented. How insecure we feel when others are misspeaking for us, misinterpreting our motives, or talking unkindly about us behind our backs. These are forms of identity theft. The Christ who knew no sin was the one who humbled Himself to be of no reputation; yet, His nature and attributes were and are important for us to know while being transformed into His likeness. How easily we spout: "to be like Jesus," when we must first learn who He really is. Then we are better skilled to share of His goodness with others. Could He trust us to be true ambassadors of His nature, His goodness, His love? Who do we say that He is? Deeper still, who do we privately think He is? Is the thief still at work in our minds, distorting His true identity from us?

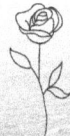
I am the light of the world. The person who follows Me will never live in darkness but will have the light that gives life. —*John 8:12*

Father, given opportunity to fully know You, and then to introduce You to others, is joy unspeakable. Grace us to portray You as the true Messiah and not a religious facsimile. Amen.

Reflection:

Coming Home

The journey can be long when pain, loss, or heartache blurs our vision. Maps are difficult to follow; directions make no sense. The road is strange and long because it's a new one yet traveled. Scenery is different. Faces have either changed or they are not perceived as they once were. All we have are questions: primarily, "What are You up to, Lord?"

Jesus came to reveal Himself to us. Though pain and heartache seem way off the main road we thought we'd take, He has a purpose. It remains true that He wants us to know Him more. To come home to Him and to have His life, His joy, and His presence. Nothing else compares.

He is the defining word on who Father God is and what Father's heart is working in us. His ways are not our ways; therefore He can be misunderstood. Modern ways of communication can blur our vision in similar ways. Emailing or text messaging does not convey our tone of voice, nor does the one receiving the message understand clearly. If we try to relate to our Lord in what compares to an electronic missive, we may fail to interpret His words and meaning. That vacant relational space yields the opportunity for misunderstanding. He works all things together for good; but try transmitting that on a text message, when adversity breaks the heart, and watch what response comes. Without Holy Spirit conveying His tone of voice, His tender care, His unsurpassable love towards His children, He comes off as hopeless as religion.

Jesus healed the man on the Sabbath, and that pushed His enemies over the top. Because this defied their religious beliefs, they decided to kill Him. (Mark 3:1-6) Jesus was habitually embroiled in conflict—that is, with the religious ones—but not with the pagan. Religion was and is His arch enemy. Behind religion is the great deceiver who comes to bring distortion to who Jesus really is.

Millions love Jesus yet only experience Him in a limited way. Lazarus was raised from the dead, leaving the tomb while wrapped in grave clothes. (John 11:38-44) Had he been left wrapped tight in bonds of religion, he would never have walked in true freedom. Alive, but not living. Religion gives an impression of Christ, yet it vaccinates you from experiencing the real.

Thus, we must discern by reading the map that guides us home to the Lord's presence. The roads homeward can appear misleading, sometimes threatening to be treacherous and dark. But as the Spirit of Truth leads the way, He will invite us to enjoy the loving presence of our God. He is the one who has promised to fill every vacuum, every void, every empty heart, to fill every absence with Himself. That is home.

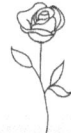 Let us then with confidence draw near to the throne of grace, that we may receive mercy and find grace to help in time of need. —*Hebrews 4:16*

Father, we long for home. Home with You is intimate communion, a glorious union between Bridegroom and Bride. Our trials and pains drive us to the realization of how much we need You, the only One who can fill our absences. Amen.

Reflection:

Chaperone

Mama always said I was not a 'cry-baby' but a 'why-baby.' Early in my young life, I believed that if I could just understand 'why' something was the way it was, I could have peace. This mindset never served me well. In fact it led to more anxiety. I did not know everything, nor could I always understand everything. I needed the One who did.

A few years back, the Spirit of God reminded me: *"Be anxious for nothing."* (Philippians 4:6 NKJV) Being assured I needed a revisit, I heard Him say, *"Look up the word 'nothing.'"* I admit I chuckled for I imagined 'nothing' to read 'nothing.' The definition I read surprised me: "not a single thing." What an impact that definition had as it led me to ask: "Not even that, Lord?" *"Not even **that**,"* He said (implying whatever 'that' is). Lessons were repeated as He taught me that truth many times since.

Losses, disappointments, and heartaches laid my soul bare for the absence of peace. That absence yielded anxiety which left me in much unrest. Many of those 'single things' took up residence in my mind—and failed to pay rent, as some say. Jesus said it clearly: "Are you weary, carrying a heavy burden? Come to Me. I will refresh your life, for I am your oasis. Simply join your life with mine. Learn my ways and you'll discover that I'm gentle, humble, easy to please. You will find refreshment and rest in Me. For all that I require of you will be pleasant and easy to bear." (Matthew 11:28-30 TPT)

He promises that His yoke is easy and His burden is light; that is, 'easy to bear.' "But, Lord!?!?! How can I manage to walk in this rest when my heart has been so overwhelmed? I don't feel safe within my own emotions. I have put myself out here on my own, and I feel lost. These thoughts trouble me with the 'whys' screeching in the dark places of my soul. I admit it: my mind, my will, and my emotions need a chaperone!"

Left to ourselves, we can get into much trouble. When chaperoned by the Spirit of God, as our daily guide into all truth, we are safe. Even as a youngster, I balked at our youth gatherings being assigned chaperones. After all, we thought we had everything under control, not understanding just how much trouble we could get into without supervision. The more I became acquainted with the fruit of my flesh and its desires to step outside the boundaries, the more I volunteered to be chaperoned!

In trying to heal ourselves, wasting time and mental anguish trying to understand the 'whys' of life, we become exhausted. Moses had spent enough time in the absence of his chaperone, being persuaded how much he needed Him.

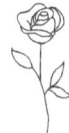 Then Moses said, 'If You don't personally go with us, don't make us leave this place. —*Exodus 33:15 NLT*

Father, I will never outgrow the need for a chaperone. Lead me. Guide me. Teach me. Heal me. Grace me to welcome Your wizsdom as well as Your comfort. Walking hand-in-hand with You through the trials of life yoke me to the One who knows answers to all the 'whys.' Help me to trust Your plan for my life, even if I don't understand. Amen.

Reflection:

Deliverance

God's ways are like the deep waters. They cannot be understood nor can they be trafficked without His guidance. He knows ways that we know not of. The waters seem great, powerful, and overwhelming, if we try to navigate them ourselves...

"Your road led through the sea," (Psalm 77:19 NLT) Leading the children of Israel into and through the great sea was unfathomable to the natural mind. Yet, He led the way, and it was the way to safety for His people.

We cannot know God's ways of deliverance. They are unknown to us; or sometimes we do not understand the greater plan allowed through His permission. "Your pathway through the mighty waters—a pathway no one knew was there!" Father God demonstrated His power with storm clouds, thunder, and lightning. He led His people by way of His chosen vessels: Moses and Aaron. The Israelites, like a flock of sheep, were led to freedom.

God will again come to the aid of His people. Though His responses may seem delayed, He has never left us abandoned. We are to remember His guiding footprints, though hidden from natural sight, were made available just at the time when His plan would be fulfilled. This same God knows of our losses, the absences of loved ones, the plight of lost provisions, the threats of declining health: the dark nights of the soul.

What lies on the other side of those daunting walls of water, positioned over the dry ocean floor, is His to determine. "Your road led through the sea," remains our hope. He is the one who leads. Though they were and are "mighty waters," there will always be His pathways "no one knew was there." Because He knows all things and His ways are higher than ours.

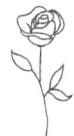

> For My thoughts are not your thoughts, neither are your ways My ways, declares the Lord. For as the heavens are higher than the earth, so are My ways higher than your ways and My thoughts higher than your thoughts...
> —Isaiah 55:8-9 ESV

Father, when the walls surround us—whatever they might be—when the enemy lurks from all sides—when fear wants to dictate our future—You remain our Deliverer! Lead us through the seas of life. Show us Your pathway, even the one we did not know was there—yet opened up just for us. The reader and I seek You as the Answer. An altar is prepared before us as we lay every burden, every yoke, every heartache at Your feet. Great is Your faithfulness to prepare a road that "no one knew was there" — yet it was. Amen

Reflection:

www.ingramcontent.com/pod-product-compliance
Lightning Source LLC
Chambersburg PA
CBHW050818090426
42737CB00021B/3427